Lecture Notes in Computer Science 6693

Commenced Publication in 1973
Founding and Former Series Editors:
Gerhard Goos, Juris Hartmanis, and Jan van Leeuwen

T0074269

José Bravo   Ramón Hervás
Vladimir Villarreal (Eds.)

Ambient Assisted Living

Third International Workshop, IWAAL 2011
Held at IWANN 2011
Torremolinos-Málaga, Spain, June 8-10, 2011
Proceedings

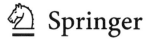 Springer

Volume Editors

José Bravo
Ramón Hervás
Castilla-La Mancha University, MAmI Research Lab
Paseo de la Universidad, 4, 13071 Ciudad Real, Spain
E-mail: {jose.bravo, ramon.hervas}@uclm.es

Vladimir Villarreal
Technological University of Panama
Panama, Republic of Panama
E-mail: vladimir.villarreal@utp.ac.pa

ISSN 0302-9743   e-ISSN 1611-3349
ISBN 978-3-642-21302-1   e-ISBN 978-3-642-21303-8
DOI 10.1007/978-3-642-21303-8
Springer Heidelberg Dordrecht London New York

Library of Congress Control Number: 2011927855

CR Subject Classification (1998): H.5.2-3, J.3, J.4, K.4.2, C.2

LNCS Sublibrary: SL 3 – Information Systems and Application, incl. Internet/Web
and HCI

Typesetting: Camera-ready by author, data conversion by Scientific Publishing Services, Chennai, India

Printed on acid-free paper

Springer is part of Springer Science+Business Media (www.springer.com)

Preface

AAL is an initiative supported by the EU Commission through a Joint Programme aiming to enhance the quality of life of elderly people living in their own homes. Motivated by the growing aging population in the world (and specifically in Europe), this initiative pursues to guarantee the quality of life of elderly people by using information and communication technologies (ICT) accessible through simple and natural users' interactions.

Aspects like e-health, inclusion, mobility, risks prevention, frailty, fall detection and revention, among others, are in the research agenda of this area. In addition, industry should get involved in providing assistive products that address elderly people's needs, a big potential market which, in general, has good economic resources in the western world.

The International Workshop on Ambient Assisted Living (IWAAL), through its three editions, promotes knowledge sharing and collaboration among researchers in the AAL field. In this third edition, 30 papers were presented, grouped in the following sections: Mobile Solutions, Smart and Wireless Sensors, Applications for Cognitive Impairments, e-Health, Methodologies, Brain–Computer Interfaces, Frameworks and Platforms.

In addition this edition had active participation from Spanish associations and platforms for AAL. We appreciate very much their efforts in addressing aging problems like Alzheimer disease, dementia and other cognitive impairments. We want to remark that the work of these platforms, governmental agencies and relatives in the daily caring activities of elderly people is very valuable. The attendance of representatives from these collectives to the workshop was very fruitful and encouraged the creation of collaborative research consortiums in future AAL calls of the European Union.

Finally, we would like to thank to the IWANN organization for the opportunity of organizing a new edition of the IWAAL workshop with their conference.

June 2011

José Bravo
Ramón Hervás
Vladimir Villarreal

Organization

General Chair

José Bravo   Castilla-La Mancha University, Spain

Organizing Committee

Jesús Fontecha	Castilla-La Mancha University (Spain)
Nadia Gámez	University of Malaga (Spain)
Isabel Diezma	Castilla-La Mancha University (Spain)
Alvaro Araujo Pinto	Polytechnic University of Madrid (Spain)

Program Committee

Xavier Alaman	Autonomous University of Madrid (Spain)
Mariano Alcañiz	Polytechnic University of Valencia (Spain)
Alvaro Araujo	Polytechnic University of Madrid (Spain)
Maria T. Arredondo	Polytechnic University of Madrid (Spain)
Rosa I. Arriaga	Georgia Tech (USA)
Juan Botia	Murcia University (Spain)
Jose Bravo - Chair	Castilla-La Mancha University (Spain)
Yan Cai	Carnegie Mellon University (USA)
Luck Chen	University of Ulster (UK)
Hariton Costing	University of Medicine and Pharmacy, Iasi (Romania)
Jesus Favela	CICESE (Mexico)
Lidia Fuentes	Malaga University (Spain)
Begoña Garcia	Deusto University (Spain)
Sergio Guillen	ITACA (Spain)
Ramon Hervas	Castilla-La Mancha University (Spain)
Robert Istepanian	Kingston University (UK)
Rui Jose	University of Minho (Portugal)
Martin Llamas	University of Vigo (Spain)
Diego Lopez-De-Ipiña	Deusto University (Spain)
Oscar Mayora	Create Net (Italy)
Rene Meier	Trinity College Dublin (Ireland)
Sofia Moreno Perez	eVIA (Spain)

Chris Nugent	University of Ulster (UK)
Marcela Rodriguez	Baja California University (Mexico)
Mario Romero	Georgia Tech (USA)
Inaki Vazquez	Deusto University (Spain)
Elena Villalba	CDTI (Spain)
Vladimir Villarreal	Technological University of Panama (Panama)

Additional Reviewers

Unai Aguilera
Aitor Almedia
Angel G. Andrade
Jesús Fontecha
Diego Gachet
Nadia Gámez
Juan P. García-Vázquez
Pau Giner
Francisco Moya
Pablo Orduña
Pere Tuset
Felix J. Villanueva

Table of Contents

3. e-Health

4. Smart and Wireless Sensors

5. Applied Technologies, Frameworks and Platforms

6. Methodologies and Brain Interfaces

Remote Monitoring and Fall Detection: Multiplatform Java Based Mobile Applications

Miguel A. Laguna and Javier Finat

GIRO and MoBiVAP Research Groups, University of Valladolid, Campus M. Delibes,
47011 Valladolid, Spain
mlaguna@infor.uva.es, jfinat@agt.uva.es

Abstract. Life quality of dependent persons is associated with personal autonomy and mobility, between others parameters. But the development of mobile applications for autonomy support is a challenging activity. Some of the challenges are the diversity of target platforms (including display sizes, keypads or tactile screens variations in each platform), and the limits in memory size, processing resources, battery duration, etc. For these reasons, a software product line (SPL) approach can provide a considerable advantage in mobile application development. This article presents a SPL that makes possible the remote monitoring of dependent people to facilitate their autonomy. Wireless sensors allow real-time information such as heart rate or oxygen saturation level to be controlled. Risk situations, including fall detection, critical in elderly persons who live alone, can also be detected. In the SPL approach, only the required features are incorporated in each concrete product (avoiding the device overload with a resource-costly extensive solution). The article presents an Android/Symbian based SPL architecture, using Bluetooth wireless sensors connected to a Smartphone. The mobile system is able to detect alarm situations and is remotely connected to a central system, aimed for its use in elderly residences.

Keywords: remote monitoring, fall detection, mobile application.

1 Introduction

The mobility of dependent people can come into conflict with frequent monitoring of health parameters under medical supervision and with risk detection. The increased costs of care and the geographic dispersion favor the deployment of personalized health services based on low cost ubiquitous systems, accessible to more people while reducing the medical costs. Consequently, one of the most interesting applications of mobile devices is the development of systems that increase the personal autonomy. These technologies have generated huge expectations but we should ensure that their costs are reasonable. The key point is that personalization of each application to the (person/sensors/mobile device) combination can be unaffordable in terms of cost and development time. To make things worse, multiple platforms for mobile devices are appearing and evolving continuously (and several display sizes, color depth and variations in keypads or tactile screens can share the same platform). For these reasons we are working in a set of projects aimed to apply the product line paradigm of software development to the specific case of customizable mobile systems.

J. Bravo, R. Hervás, and V. Villarreal (Eds.): IWAAL 2011, LNCS 6693, pp. 1–8, 2011.

Software product lines (SPL) combine systematic development and the reuse of coarse-grained components that include the common and variable parts of the product line [3]. Tough successful, this approach is complex and requires a great effort by the companies that take it on. The research we carry out in the GIRO group aims to simplify the change from a conventional development process towards one that benefits from the product line advantages. For this reason, we proposed to use the standard UML package merge relationship to represent the SPL architecture variations with conventional CASE and IDE tools [8]. We have used that approach with several mobile systems. The requirements for a remote monitoring SPL were presented in [7]. This paper reports the practical experiences in the implementation of this SPL for remote monitoring systems for dependent people, using a combination of sensors, Android and Symbian based mobile devices and a central server that can be consulted in real time from anywhere by medical personnel using a standard Internet browser.

A distinctive characteristic is the use of conventional CASE and IDE tools, a precondition imposed by our goal of simplifying the adoption of the SPL paradigm. In particular, we have used Java/Eclipse and the Android and Symbian platforms for the implementation of the remote monitoring SPL. Only a specific plug-in is required to handle the feature models and the configuration process, distinctive of the SPL approach. The personnel involved vary from postgraduate students to undergraduates finishing their term projects but, in any case, not specialists in SPL development.

The rest of the article is organized as follows: Section 2 briefly presents the technique used for the SPL design and implementation, based on the package merge relationship of UML. Section 3 is devoted to the description of the remote monitoring SPL. In Section 4 the related work is analyzed and, finally, Section 5 concludes the article and outlines future work.

2   Software Product Lines and the Package Merge Relationship

The specific SPL techniques are aimed to handle variability and traceability at each abstraction level of the product line. The product line development requires models that represent the SPL variability and a mechanism to obtain the configuration of features that represent the best combination of variants for each specific application. Additionally, the optional features must be connected with the related variation points of the architectural models that implement the SPL through traceability links. This explicit connection allows the automatic instantiation of the SPL generic architecture into each specific application. This is derived from the complete architecture selecting or not each optional feature, fulfilling the concrete set of functional and non-functional requirements. The selected feature sub-model, through traceability relationships, guides the composition of the pre-existing code packages. The precondition for the success of this process is the existence of traceability links from features to design and from design to implementation.

Our solution to this problem [8] consist of expressing the SPL variability of UML models using the package merge relationship, defined in the UML infrastructure meta-model. This mechanism permits a clear traceability between feature and UML models to be established. The technique consists of associating a package to each optional feature, so that all the necessary elements that model the feature remain located in a package (maintaining the UML meta-model unchanged and separating both variability levels). The resulting package model is hierarchical, reflecting the feature diagram structure. Considering each pair of related packages, the dependent package can only be included if the base package is also selected. Therefore, the application to SPL consists of building the architectural model (including structural – class diagrams-, behavioral -use cases-, and dynamic –interaction diagram- models) starting from a base package that gathers the common SPL aspects. Then, each variability point detected in the feature diagram originates a package, connected through a merge relationship with its parent package. When each product is derived, these packages will be combined or not, according to the selected feature configuration.

Additionally, using C# partial classes (or an adapted version of Java) organized in packages, a direct connection between design and code can be established. Therefore a one-to-one relationship from features to design and from design to implementation is recorded. As an added value, the package structure of the code for each final product of the SPL can be obtained automatically (and passed to the compiler) from the features configuration [8].

To achieve this, making the technique readily accessible to developers, we use the FeatureIDE plug-in for Eclipse [6] that allows using Java classes in a similar way to the native C# partial classes. This can be a good solution for mobile devices that use Java as their preferred language. In the case of our SPL, we have designed a platform independent architecture and subsequently we can implement different platform specific SPL designs for C# (Windows Mobile platform) and Java (Symbian and Android platforms). The Java version requires two different implementations, due to the characteristics of the Android platform that do not use the standard Java ME facilities, in particular the standard user interface libraries. We present in this article the details of the Android and Symbian versions of the SPL.

3 Multiplatform Remote Monitoring Product Line

The product line was planned initially with independence of any particular platform and the requirements were presented in [7], together with a first prototype, developed in C# for Windows Mobile devices. However, due to the greater presence in the market of the Android and Symbian Smartphones, we decided to implement the complete SPL using Java for these platforms.

Apart from continuous monitoring, other eventual situations can be considered. The possibility of cancelling an alarm signal or manually raising one (*Panic Button*) should be included in most systems. On the other hand, in aged people, accidental falls represent a frequent risk, that can be detected with an accelerometer based sensor and an adequate algorithm. An experimental prototype was developed with a set of requirements, validated by the medical staff of a senior citizens' residence that collaborates with us in developing monitoring systems. This experimental system used a well known gamepad as accelerometer connected via Bluetooth with a workstation (no libraries were available to connect a windows mobile device in a simple way). The .NET platform and C # were used to develop the system, due to the ease of integration with the available libraries. The experimental version was intended for home scenarios (or a small residence), since the limits are defined by the Bluetooth connection range (a maximum theoretical distance of 100 meters, much less in practical situations). The results were satisfactory both in fall detection and false positive rejection [9]. This experience has been very useful for the integration of the *WiTilt* sensor in the remote monitoring SPL. The WiTilt sensor is a professional tri-axial accelerometer with a standard communication protocol accessible from any mobile device using Java o C# languages and common Bluetooth libraries [16].

Finally, a set of platform related decisions must be taken. Some important differences concern device types (smart or conventional phones, PDAs, etc.) and operating systems (Windows mobile, Android, Symbian tactile and keypad based devices, etc.).

These requirements lead to an implementation with a hierarchical package structure. The SPL base package support the continuous monitoring of patients. To prevent failures, the right operation of sensors is verified in the mobile device. If local or remote validations fail, alert signals are raised. Once validated, the sequence of values is analyzed, comparing the read values with the intended range as set by health professionals. A module allows rules to be configured that use customizable calculations to detect risk situations alert. Alarms can be generated in the presence of critical values for original or calculated values, and then this information is sent (combined with the last available location is the positioning feature is also selected) to the central system. The elapsed time from the moment of detection until the alarm is sent allows the person to cancel the alarm if it is a false positive. The system shows also locally each sensor's data and risk state.

The generic positioning package must be combined with the GPS or Wi-Fi variants (or both), to get the patient location directly in devices equipped with built-in GPS or using an approximate position obtained from the existing indoor Wi-Fi antennas. Other packages add the fall detection or the remote configuration features.

The distributed architecture of the system has been designed and implemented following the scheme of Figure 1. The data are collected by the mobile device and sent to the central system using a Web service via http. If a situation reflects abnormal parameters or a possible fall, the mobile device indicates to the patient the problem and after a few seconds an alarm is generated to be sent to a central system using the Web service. The Web service saves the received data in a Database that is used by a typical Web application, accessible from any Internet browser. The coordinates that the mobile application sends to the Central System are used with the Google Maps API to represent the position of the monitored person inside the residence (or its outdoor position).

The architecture fulfils usual constraints relative to customized configuration, the use of Web services for communications between the mobile device and the central system, and security in data transmission. Security in Bluetooth transmission is granted by associating the sensor to a unique device (password required) during configuration phase. On the other hand, secure Web services are similar to the HTTPS standard.

Due to the experience of the development team and the advantages of using the enhanced Visual Studio/FMT platform, the first prototypes were initially developed using PDAs and Smartphones that support Windows Mobile. Java/Eclipse and the

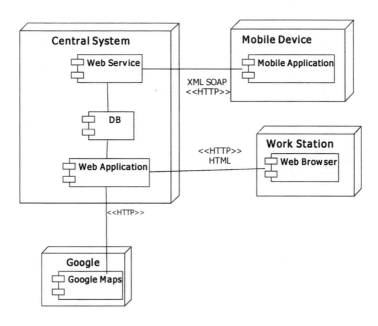

Fig. 1. Deployment diagram of the generic monitoring system

FeatureIde plug-in have been used to develop the alternative implementations for the Android and Symbian platforms. The Java versions have been developed in parallel for the two platforms. Both have a common part that is basically the domain model but, however, each platform uses different user interface frameworks. The support libraries for Bluetooth communications are also specific for each platform. In the Symbian version we use standard Java ME to implement a simple interface. In the Android version, the native activities and XML definition of the user interfaces are used. The techniques used for adding optional parts to the user interface are based on dynamic addition of widgets. An array of widgets (or menus) can be complemented dynamically using the optional code incorporated in each package. Figure 2 shows an example of the user interface for a product configuration in Android.

In both platforms, health parameters, such as heart rate and oxygen saturation, have been evaluated and controlled by software using the data sent from a commercial wireless sensor. Also the GPS and indoor Wi-Fi positioning module for integrated devices and Bluetooth/Wi-Fi communication features have been implemented. Wi-Fi/3G is used to communicate directly with the central system using a Web service. If there is no Wi-Fi connectivity, alerts can be sent using SMS messages directly to a configurable telephone number, covering the risk situations when the Internet connection is unavailable. In the case of Symbian, an additional application developed in C++ must be included, due to Java ME restrictions.

Several configurations of the SPL have been deployed for different Symbian (Nokia 5800) and Android (Samsung Galaxy, HTC Hero) mobile devices. The sensor used (Figure 2) was a Nonin Bluetooth pulsi-oximeter [12] that provides heart-rate and oxygen saturation values. The fall detection package has been developed for the

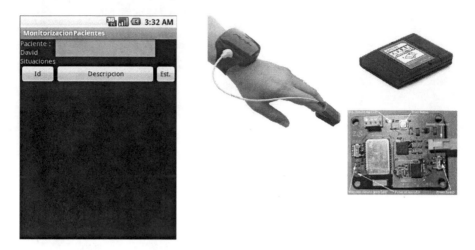

Fig. 2. Main form of a configuration in Android, the pulsi-oximeter sensor, and the tri-axial accelerometer (external and internal view) used in the SPL

Java platforms implementing the algorithm presented in [9] using Bluetooth communication with the WiTilt sensor (Figure 2). Bluetooth communication and GPS positioning are managed using the platform native libraries.

Finally, Figure 3 shows the user interface that medical personnel uses to monitor the location of a patient (using the Google Maps API), the alarms raised, and the graphical representation of the monitored parameters (in the example, the oxygen saturation). The use of standard SOAP based Web services to communicate with the central station has the advantage that no changes are needed in the server when an application is configured for a new mobile platform. Also in the server, the monitored data is made persistent using a database. Finally, a conventional Web application makes the data available to medical staff using an Internet browser. The Web service and the Web application for monitoring were developed using ASP/.NET and SQL Server under Windows but is used transparently by the three mobile platforms.

4   Related Work

There are many works that use mobile devices and sensors for remote monitoring [10] [15], including commercial solutions [5]. Most of these works are ad hoc solutions, valid for concrete platforms and sensors. However, we are mainly interested in generic or configurable approaches comparable to ours. Some of these works provide design patterns and generic tools for SPL design and configuration in the mobile domain. For example, in [4] some architecture patterns were specified in a platform independent and adaptable way. Also generic, [11] present a requirement analysis for mobile middleware, based on a product line approach, including mobility concerns that should be addressed to customize the compliant platforms versions.

Changing the approach, Anastasopoulos [2] uses Aspect Oriented Programming (AOP) as an alternative for building Java ME product lines. The same AOP technique is used by [1] in the context of an industrial mobile product line.

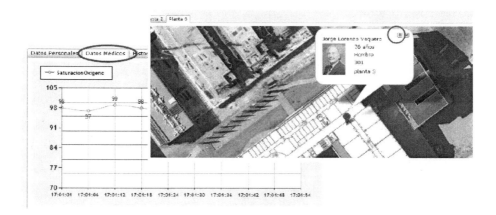

Fig. 3. Generic view of the implemented architecture of the SPL monitoring system and the user interface as seen by the medical personnel

These proposals need specific techniques and languages that are not usual in a typical software company. Though these solutions are valid, the learning of new modeling or implementation techniques and the need of specialized CASE and IDE tools represent barriers for the adoption of the approach of product lines in many organizations; we therefore believe that the UML/conventional IDE solution presented here improves the abovementioned proposals.

5 Conclusions

In this work the viability of a product line development approach to customizable mobile system has been shown. The use of the package merge relationship and partial classes (adapting the Java language) enables the automated generation of each product from the features configuration. Furthermore, the use of conventional CASE and IDE tools can simplify the adoption of this paradigm, avoiding the need of specific tools and techniques as in previous alternatives.

The approach has been successfully applied to the design and implementation of a product line in the domain of remote monitoring, implemented with mobile devices. The remote monitoring systems can facilitate the autonomy of dependent people. Heart rate or oxygen saturation data are obtained with wireless sensors. Risk situations (deduced from those values or from a fall suspicion) can also be detected. The diversity of individual situations and the resource limitations of mobile devices favor the use of the SPL paradigm. In the context of a senior citizen residence, we use a combination of sensors/mobile devices with a monitoring central server accessible from any Internet browser.

The personnel involved were last year undergraduate students and recent graduates. Some of these had professional experience but they were not specialists in SPL development. The orientation of the author was enough to accomplish the feature modeling, the only specific SPL technique used during the development process.

Acknowledgments

This work has been funded by the Spanish MICIINN, through the ADISPA (BIA2009-14254-C02-01) and TIN2008-05675 projects.

References

1. Alves, V., Matos Jr., P., Cole, L., Borba, P., Ramalho, G.: Extracting and Evolving Mobile Games Product Lines. In: Obbink, H., Pohl, K. (eds.) SPLC 2005. LNCS, vol. 3714, pp. 70–81. Springer, Heidelberg (2005)
2. Anastasopoulos, M., Muthig, D.: An evaluation of aspect-oriented programming as a product line implementation technology. In: Dannenberg, R.B., Krueger, C. (eds.) ICOIN 2004 and ICSR 2004. LNCS, vol. 3107, pp. 141–156. Springer, Heidelberg (2004)
3. Bosch, J.: Design & Use of Software Architectures. In: Adopting and Evolving a Product-Line Approach. Addison-Wesley, Reading (2000)
4. Cho, H., Yang, J.S.: Architecture patterns for mobile games product lines. In: International Conference on Advanced Communication Technology, ICACT, pp. 118–122 (2008)
5. Ericsson Mobile Health, http://www.ericsson.com/hr/ict_solutions/e-health/emh
6. FeatureIde: Eclipse-Plugin for Feature-Oriented Software Development. Otto-von-Guericke-Universität Magdeburg (2011), http://www.fosd.de/fide
7. Laguna, M.A., Finat, J., González, J.A.: Remote Health Monitoring: A Customizable Product Line Approach. In: Omatu, S., Rocha, M.P., Bravo, J., Fernández, F., Corchado, E., Bustillo, A., Corchado, J.M. (eds.) IWANN 2009. LNCS, vol. 5518, pp. 727–734. Springer, Heidelberg (2009)
8. Laguna, M.A., González-Baixauli, B., Marqués, J.M.: Seamless Development of Software Product Lines: Feature Models to UML Traceability. In: GPCE 2007 (2007)
9. Laguna, M.A., Tirado, M.J., Finat, J., Marqués, J.M.: Fall Detection Systems: A Solution Based on Low Cost Sensors. In: Proceedings of ICSOFT 2010 (2010)
10. Lubrin, E., Lawrence, E., Navarro, K.F.: Wireless Remote Healthcare Monitoring with Motes. In: International Conference on Mobile Business (ICMB 2005), pp. 235–241 (2005)
11. Morais, Y., Burity, T., Elias, G.: Towards a mobile middleware product line: A requirement analysis. In: ITNG 2010 - 7th International Conference on Information Technology: New Generations (2010)
12. Nonin, Pulse Oximetry Monitoring (2011), http://www.nonin.com/PulseOximetry
13. Salva, A., Bolibar, I., Pera, G., Arias, C.: Incidence and consequences of falls among elderly people living in the community. Med. Clin. (Barc) 122(5), 172–176 (2004)
14. Sochos, P., Philippow, I., Riebisch, M.: Feature-oriented development of software product lines: Mapping feature models to the architecture. In: Weske, M., Liggesmeyer, P. (eds.) NODe 2004. LNCS, vol. 3263, pp. 138–152. Springer, Heidelberg (2004)
15. Tocino, A.V., Gutiérrez, J.J.A., Navia, I.Á., Peñalvo, F.J.G., Castrejón, E.P., Giner, J.R.G.-B.: Personal Health Monitor. In: Damiani, E., Jeong, J., Howlett, R.J., Jain, L.C. (eds.) New Directions in Intelligent Interactive Multimedia Systems and Services - 2. SCI, vol. 226, pp. 465–475. Springer, Heidelberg (2009)
16. WiTilt, SparkFun Electronics (2011), http://www.sparkfun.com/products/8563

Results of Mobility and Obstacles Detection of an Experimental Three-Legged Prototype for Blind and Deafblind People

J. Alberto Garcia and Javier Poncela

Institute of Innovation for Human Wellbeing, Severo Ochoa 16-20, 29590, Business Park, Málaga, Spain
{algarcia,jponcela}@i2bc.es
http://www.i2bc.es

Abstract. Blindness or visual impairments may result in a loss of personal autonomy, an important disability when its onset is related to ageing. In this paper we present an ongoing project which is developing a guide robot with the aim of helping people with limited vision in their daily life ("InviGBot"), improving their mobility in the street. The main design criteria have been the simplicity of use and a reduced cost, so that it can be afforded by most users. One of the most innovative elements of InviGBot are its three articulated legs, which provide the capability of easily avoiding obstacles. Thus, it only requires six servomotors (two per leg), which represents two elements fewer than usually required for four-leg designs.

Keywords: blind guide, tripod robot, obstacle avoidance, ultrasound sensor, user centered design.

1 Introduction

Personal autonomy of visual impaired people normally decreases along time, becoming an important disability when ageing [1]. In Spain there are nearly one million visually impaired people, and half of them are not satisfied with the available helps [2]. This figure shows the high dissatisfaction with the technological solutions that support mobility outdoors. Besides, in most cases, they are too expensive for the average citizen. Data shows the need for a cheap and effective technological solution.

The field of robotics has shown special interest for years in tackling these challenges. Researchers have mainly been concerned with solving technical difficulties to create mobile robots for effectively guiding blind people [3]. Since 1965 there exist projects for guiding blind people using new technologies. The Russell Pathsounder [4] device was the first to use ultrasound sensors with this aim. This device consisted of two ultrasonic transducers placed around the neck of the user. Its mission was reporting the distance to an obstacle, differentiating between three thresholds with a series of clicks. The problem of this device was that the person had to orient his torso to detect an obstacle in the desired direction. More recently, the "Guide Dog Robot" project [5] it's one of the first references similar to our

J. Bravo, R. Hervás, and V. Villarreal (Eds.): IWAAL 2011, LNCS 6693, pp. 9–16, 2011.

objectives. This robot, developed in the Engineering Laboratory of Tsukuba Science Center, was a mobile robot that used both ultrasonic sensors and cameras. It created a map with intersections and distances between the robot and the user; the robot speed could be adapted according to the user speed. The processed information was transmitted to the user through a voice synthesizer. Even so, this robot wasn't designed to detect obstacles and to avoid them, in addition it was too heavy to be carried by a person.

Today, such a robot should move smoothly through dynamic environments, such as streets or shopping malls. Solutions require more intelligent and context-aware robots, which can adapt to any topography and objects distribution of the environment [6]. Even with plenty of research to find a clever technological solution for guiding the blind, the prototypes created haven't reached the real market. In comparison, basic technological devices such as electronic canes, based on different sensor technologies (ultrasound, GPS, RFID, etc.), are available today. However, the dog guide still remains the most popular solution, even though it has known problems such as incompatibility with allergies, social rejection, high cost in maintenance and education, etc. [7].

2   First Prototype

Now, advanced microelectronic devices are available at low prices. The target of the InviGBot project is to reach a mobile robotic platform suitable to guide a person in street environments, such as sidewalks routes, always keeping in mind the final price of the robot. It should overcome small obstacles, such as steps, and not only reporting and avoiding them. This requirement makes us choose the use of a legged-based mechanism, and, then, to propose a tripod structure for the movement of the system. The reasons are three-fold: less material to waste on legs, less number of motors and, because of it, less consumption of the entire system.

Along this ongoing research, we have already developed a robotic prototype that detects obstacles found in the path, avoids them, and informs the user about the type of barrier detected (e.g. step or wall). Its walking direction is always forward; if it finds a corner it will turn away from it, but it will never go backwards. These characteristics allow it to basically guide both blind and deafblind people in an innovative way.

The system functionality is organized in modules, which are managed as peripheral subsystems connected to a central control unit. The responsibilities of these modules are: providing energy suitable to each module, detecting obstacles, interfacing with

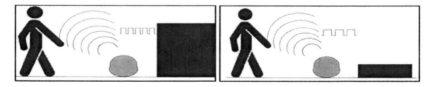

Fig. 1. Codification used to inform about detected obstacles; (left) "high obstacle", (right) "low obstacle"

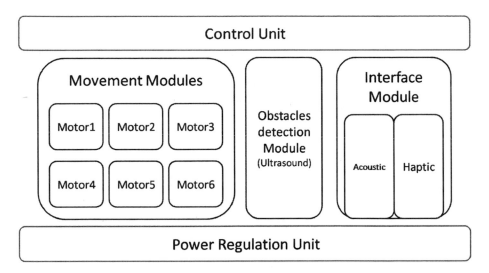

Fig. 2. System Modules

the user and executing the movements. Each of them has been designed and programmed using matured technologies of sensors and actuators.

Power is provided by a 12V/5000mAh Lion polymer battery, which ensures a minimum estimated operating time of 8 hours. The control of the system is performed by a TI MSP430F169 microprocessor; it has been programmed in assembler to meet the memory and performance requirements.

To identify obstacles we use an ultrasonic sensor located in the front of the robot leg. It scans forward a 30° sonic cone (see Fig.3.a) after each step and checks that the path is clear. The scanner uses a 40KHz signal, which is the frequency of highest sensitivity of the sensor. The height of the obstacle is measured by rising the front leg.

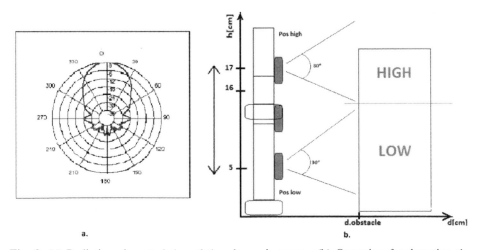

Fig. 3. (a) Radiation characteristics of the ultrasonic sensor. (b) Operation for detecting the height.

If it doesn't detect any obstacle in the higher position, the obstacle is assumed to be "low"; otherwise the obstacle is classified as "high." The range of heights classified as "low" is 3-16cm and it is above 16 cm for a "high" classification (Fig. 3.b). In this way, the same sensor can be used to increase the area of vertical coverage.

Information on the height of detected obstacles is provided to the user via acoustic signals and, optionally, vibrations on a wearable device. The frequencies are 1 KHz for low obstacles and 2 KHz for higher ones. Communication with the vibrator device is carried out in FM.

2.1 Walking Pattern

The movements of this prototype is realized with three legs. Only six analog servomotors are required, which represents two fewer than on quadruped robots. This makes it possible to decrease the cost of the materials and the power consumption. This design feature allows for effective movement on surfaces such as sand or stone, where the use of wheels poses more difficulties.

To attempt to hold this advantage and achieving a walking algorithm more simple, we have designed the structure with one toehold in the center of its body. This toehold doesn't provide of any extra functionality to help the forward movement, it's only used to having the third toehold, necessary for a correct balance [8]. It's composed by one stick with a free ball at the bottom, it hasn't been considered as another leg because it doesn't have associated any actuator. In its movement of walking we can differentiate four frames: moving right, left and front legs, and repositioning of the body (the advance movement) (Fig.4). The stability of the movement is achieved via the combination of the movement of the legs and the tilting of the body on this center toehold, so that it doesn't need any accelerometer or gyroscope. The first step is used to balance its body to the left for moving the right leg, leaning on the center toehold and on the left and front legs. In the second one it balances itself to the right for

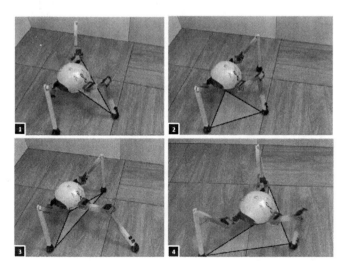

Fig. 4. Toeholds of InviGBot in its walking model

moving the left leg, leaning on the center toehold and on the right and front legs. The third step helps to stretch the front leg, having the three toeholds behind. To end, it does the final step moving all its legs simultaneously backwards, so it can advance forwards. In this final movement the center toehold is elevated for not to crash with any small obstacle. In a static analysis of the movement, the projection of the center of gravity must be within the area of the polygon that is formed with the legs that are supporting the body of the robot (Fig.4). This is the indispensable condition that prevents the robot from falling.

In order to reducing the material costs, the entire structure has been designed using the minimal number of pieces and actuators. The two side legs have two degrees of freedom: forwards-backwards, up and down. To get increase the adaptability to the terrain of a passive way and, at the same time, maintaining always the same position of the leg, it has been used a passive spring at the free joint of the leg.

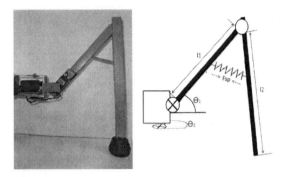

Fig. 5. Photograph (left) and schematic of the one side leg of the robot (right). It consists of two servomotors at the hip joint (represented by a circle with a cross) and two limb segments connected through a compliant passive joint (marked by an open circle).

The front leg also has two degrees of freedom: up-down and contracted-stretched. In this case it has one servomotor at the hip joint and the other one at the free joint. Such as the lateral legs as the front leg are conformed by two pieces of the same length.

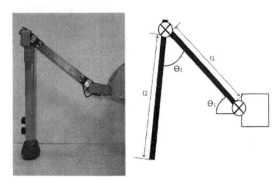

Fig. 6. Photograph (left) and schematic of the one front leg of the robot (right). It consists of two servomotors, one at the hip joint and other at the free joint (both represented by a circle with a cross).

3 Experimental Tests

The tests have been designed to verify proper operation of this prototype. These tests have checked the detection of walls with different heights and configurations (Fig. 5), as well as the user recognition of the audio signals. The speed results achieved by the robot are shown on Table 1. The movement of the robot can be improved, however it moves faster than other robots with more legs. The velocity is conditioned by the power consumption of the actuators, because the battery can't provide the required power for that. The positioning velocity of the servomotor (0.13sec/60° at no load) is

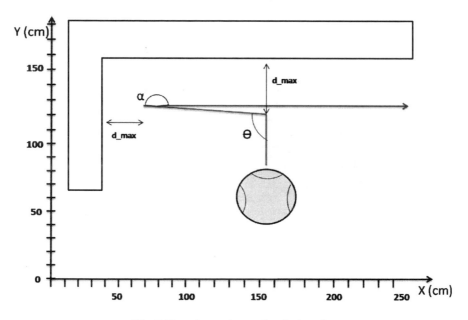

Fig. 7. Experimental test of wall obstacles

Table 1. Results values of the InviGBot prototype

Variable	Value
d_max_detection (cm)	25cm
Turn angle (Θ)	90°
Angle of reverse (α)	175°
Time to detect the obstacle's height	5.10sec
Time to turn Θ angle (from detection of obstacle to end of the turn).	7.8sec
Time to reverse (from detection of obstacle to end of the reverse).	15.7sec
d_max_vibration (cm)	150cm
Speed (m/s)	0.07m/s

other limiting factor, which affects the minimum time for the organization of the legs between movements. The distance to detect an obstacle can be adjusted by an internal potentiometer; it has been set for detection at 25 centimeters because it's the minimum necessary to turn around without touching the obstacle.

4   Conclusions

This prototype is a good first approach to the project objective, where the users can have a good context-aware approximation for getting realistic feelings about their interaction with the proposed solution. It costs around two hundred euros, which it's a low starting price. It presents three main technical problems that require to be improved: it can't detect obstacles around it to select the best direction to turn, it's too slow to guide a person in a normal walking pace and it cannot overcome any obstacle yet.

In addition to the technical objectives, the aim is achieving a high degree of psychological and economic acceptance for most people. We are carrying out the next stage: the evaluation with real end users based on the PLI [9] (People Led Innovation) model, which represents an evolution of the "user centered design" approach. The conceptual development of PLI extracts elements, techniques and experiences from other innovation methodologies related to the users' participation in design and validation processes of services and products. This methodology has already been used in the evaluation of digital technological devices in other projects [10].

We are designing an advanced prototype that seeks more and better functionalities based on additional sensors, which main idea is to propose safe sidewalks routes to transit for blind and deaf-blind people. It will include usability suggestions taken from the opinions received from users.

References

1. National Statistics Institute of Spain. Overview of disability in Spain, Madrid (2008) issn:1579-2277
2. National Statistics Institute of Spain, Madrid (2008)
3. Shoval, S., Ulrich, I., Borenstein, J.: Computerized Obstacle Avoidance Systems for the Blind and Visually Impaired. In: Teodorescu, H.N.L., Jain, L.C. (eds.) Intelligent Systems and Technologies in Rehabilitation Engineering, CRC Press, Boca Raton (2000) ISBN/ISSN: 0849301408 6
4. Russell, L.: Travel Path Sounder. In: Proceedings of Rotterdam Mobility Res. Conference, American Foundation for the Blind, New York (1965)
5. Tachi, S., Tanie, K., Komoriya, K., Abe, M.: Electrocutaneous Comunication in a Guide Dog Robot (MELDOG). IEEE Transactions on Biomedical Engineering BME-32(7) (1985)
6. Dudek, G., Jenkin, M.: Computational Principles of Mobile Robotics, 2nd edn. Cambridge University Press, Cambridge (2010) ISBN: 978-0-521-69212-0
7. Gazzano, A., Mariti, C., Sighieri, C., et al.: Survey of undesirable behaviors displayed by potential guide dogs with puppy walkers. Journal of Veterinay Behavior-Clinical Applications and Research (2008), doi:10.1016/j.jveb.2008.04.002

8. Vargas Soto, J.E.: Diseño un Robot Hexápodo Tipo Hormiga. In: Proceedings of the VIII Mexican Robotic Congress COMRob, October 19-20 (2006)
9. I2BC and SGS ICS. Reference of certification for solutions designed under the principles of technological effectiveness. I2BC Technical Report (2008)
10. Sainz, F., Madrid, R.I., Madrid, J.: Introducing co-design for digital technologies in rural areas. In: Proceedings of the NORDICHI 2010 Conference, Reykjavik, Iceland, October 18-20, pp. 769–772 (2010)

Mobile Augmented Reality Based on the Semantic Web Applied to Ambient Assisted Living

Ramón Hervás, Alberto Garcia-Lillo, and José Bravo

Castilla – La Mancha University, Paseo de la Universidad 4,
13071 Ciudad Real, Spain
ramon.hlucas@uclm.es, alberto.garcia20@alu.uclm.es,
jose.bravo@uclm.es

Abstract. This paper presents an infrastructure for supporting elderly-people needs by simple interactions with the environment through an augmented-reality perspective. We propose a general and adaptive model to transform physical information of objects in the environment into a virtual representation through accelerometers and digital compasses. The model also makes use of principles of the Semantic Web that provides context-awareness and user personalization to the proposed services. The model have been adapted to implement an application using iPhone technology and applied to illustrative problems into Ambient Assisted Living scenarios.

Keywords: Augmented reality, Mobile Computing, Ambient Intelligence, Ambient Assisted Living, Context-awareness, Semantic Web.

1 Introduction

Elderly people living alone at home need support for daily activities. For this reason, the Ambient Assisted Living (AAL) [1] initiative promotes the use of technologies for helping elderly people to maintain their autonomy, increasing their quality of life and facilitating their daily activities, but bearing in mind that it is crucial serving users in terms of usability. It is important to consider that an important number of elderly people presents disorders of memory, orientation and cognition. Cases in witch these disorders are severe need holistic attention by caregivers, however, slight cases can achieve a personal autonomy adapting technologies to the performance of their daily activities and needs.

However, choosing the correct devices for each patient is still difficult. While one person responds appropriately to a monitoring system, another may prefer a simple sound to refresh his or her memory. So, there are devices that can be adapted to the individual patient. In this sense, the chosen technology has to be unobtrusive and wireless. We propose the use of mobile devices as a common and well-known technology being aware of the difficulties to elderly people to interact with the menus and application of these devices. In this way, we are developed the mobile applications following simplicity and intuitive principles.

In fact, Mobile Health is an emergent area and it is hardly related to AAL. Several relevant works regarding to this area have been proposed in the last few years. For

J. Bravo, R. Hervás, and V. Villarreal (Eds.): IWAAL 2011, LNCS 6693, pp. 17–24, 2011.

example, several mobile-based systems to alleviate problems posed by chronic diseases such as Diabetes Mellitus [2], Alzheimer [3] and mobility disorders [4] have been developed. Not only illnesses but also common daily activities can be supported by means of mobile services, for example: shopping lists, catering, calls [5] mobile prescriptions [6] and social interactions [7].

Augmented reality applied to health is also an explored topic. For example, Breton-Lopez et al. [8] have developed a system to analyze the anxiety level by simulating a real phobia-inducing situation and generating an adapted therapy. However, augmented reality applied to AAL through mobile devices is still an area to explore.

In this paper, we present a proposal for supporting elderly people needs by simple interactions with the environment through an augmented-reality perspective. Further, we propose a generalization of these services based on a conceptual model that enable the implementation of augmented-reality applications. The model makes use of principles of Semantic Web that endow context-awareness and user personalization to the proposed services. In addition, this kind of services allows relatives and assistants making easy the supervision and management of what is happening at home and to detect incidences in an early moment.

This paper is organized into five sections. Section 2 describes the scenario of application into the AAL perspective. Section 3 presents a general model linking information to relevant elements in the environment and techniques to formalize the representation of how the user world is and infer what activities users want to do. The model also includes several general metrics to transform the information about relevant objects and their representation in an augmented-reality-based view. This model is independent of the technology to link information to a relevant element, to acquire it and the particular implementation of the augmented reality interface. Section 4 describes a particular implementation based on this model utilizing the iPhone technology and shows several real applications. Finally, Section 6 analyzes the conclusions and contributions of this paper.

2   Scenario

Elderly people living alone sometimes have a medical condition that can be neuro-degenerative and can display cognitive impairments or light behaviour disorders. As consequence, they can have troubles to perform some daily activities. It is important to contribute to the patients' ongoing improvement or maintenance in independent personal and social functioning.

In the development of this work, we follow the metaphor *how to*, that is, the environment establishes guidelines of how to perform a task whenever the user interacts with an augmented element in the user's home. We consider augmented element any object or area in the environment that has associate some information and offers a mechanism to interact with it and to share the linked information. There are multiple technologies and mechanisms to achieve these requirements; in Section 3.1 we have described some of them and justified the chosen mechanism.

Once acquired the information from an augmented element, the user receives the guidelines to perform the wanted activity. Precisely in this step appears a problem: there is not a unique relationship between an augmented element and an activity to perform. In order to disambiguate this relationship we propose to endow context-awareness to our system by means of the principles and languages of the Semantic Web. The definition of a formal context model that represents the users and their surroundings we can determine what activity they want to perform, specifically, applying the semantic axioms of the language associated to the context model and defining behavior rules that represent how the user's world works.

3 General Model for Mobile-Based Augmented Reality

This section is focused on describing the generic model that we have defined to generate augmented reality mobile applications in a general, reusable and applicable way. The developed model called Mobile Augmented-reality Model (MARM) let us transform situation of objects in real environments into an understandable language for the device. This model is independent from the specific features of mobile device; it only has a condition: the device must to be able to obtain accelerometer and digital compass data. For thit formal description, the model includes a language based on RDF[1] to define data from the real situation of the relevant objects. Based on this data and the knowledge base for each scenario, it is possible to determine which elements will be shown depending on the user needs. Also, the model defines the correlation between the device movements and the automatic adaptation of the elements in the user interface.

3.1 Interaction with Augmented Elements

The model does not impose the technology to obtain the defined information regarding to relevant elements. In this case, we chose QR codes from another alternatives as NFC technology or 2D marks. This decision was based on several reasons: (a) QR codes only need a camera in the mobile device. They don't require any kind of additional infrastructure; (b) the cost of QR codes is very low because they are sheet of paper where the codes are printed. However, NFC requires tags with integrated antenna and memory, which is more expensive than QR codes; (c) the goal of 2D marks is not code information, but it establishes a mark to situate coordinates in the user interface; and (d) NFC was rejected because it just results interesting when tag data change, but data are statics in this case.

3.2 Semantic Context Information

The use of ontological approaches in AAL brings forth several benefits and additional functionalities. The ontology formalization is the first step to exploit the benefits of this kind of formal conceptualization. In general, this formalization is a powerful mechanism for structuring, organizing and reusing knowledge. The Semantic Web provides a common framework that enables people and machines to share information, describing the semantics of concepts and services on the web and in AAL in general, and for inferring the user intention in the particular case of this proposal.

---

[1] http://www.w3.org/RDF/

Based on these premises, the information associated to augmented elements has been described through the OWL language[2] and it is part of a general context-model. The proposed model defines four taxonomical elements to be specialized: (a) User Ontology, describing the user profile, their situation and their social relationships; (b) Device Ontology, that is the formal description of the relevant devices and their characteristics, associations and dependencies; (c) Physical Environment Ontology, defining the space distribution; and (d) Service Ontology to describe the adaptive services offered to users, including the needed data to transform the sensor values with the stored elements to finally be represented in the augmented-reality-based interface. Specifically, these data are instances of the following classes: elementName (representative name of the element), elementDistance (distance between object and user), acclrmtr (height of the element in reference to the user), cmpass (degrees of the element around the user), and urlElement (OWL URI of this element).

The context model [9] and context management architecture COIVA [10] have been described in a previous document and are not our interest here; in this paper we discuss the mechanism to generate adaptive services based on augmented reality for AAL.

3.3 Matching between Reality and Virtuality

This subsection is regarding to the mechanism to transform the object information and the device sensor parameters into augmented information in the user interface. The application will recover every associated value at the object. This information is linked to a graphic component, which will appear in the display as an object representation. Finally, the mobile device will send values from compass and accelerometer to the application, so it could refresh the elements in the X-axis through the compass values and the Y-axis using accelerometer values.

3.3.1 X-Asis (Compass)

Firstly, we need to know if the object is in the camera's field of view. This is solved calculating the absolute value of distance (in degrees) between the object and compass direction. If it is lower than half of the field of view, the object is out of the display; otherwise the object is inside.

$$
pX \begin{cases} Abs(objX - cmpass) > \left(\dfrac{kDegreesVision}{2} \right): pX = \begin{cases} cmpass < 180: pX = \begin{cases} (objX > cmpass) \& (objX < (cmpass + 180)): pX = kXAxisRight \\ (objX <= cmpass) \| (objX >= (cmpass + 180)): pX = kXAxisLeft \end{cases} \\ cmpass >= 180: pX = \begin{cases} (objX < cmpass) \& (objX > (cmpass - 180)): pX = kXAxisLeft \\ (objX >= cmpass) \| (objX <= (cmpass - 180)): pX = kXAxisRight \end{cases} \end{cases} \\ Abs(objX - cmpass) <= \left(\dfrac{kDegreesVision}{2} \right): pX = (objX - cmpass) * \left(\dfrac{kWidthPixels}{kDegreesVision} \right) + \left(\dfrac{kWidthPixels}{2} \right) \end{cases}
$$

$$(1)$$

$$(2)$$

In case the object has to be shown inside the screen, the equation 2 returns its position in pixels (pX), where $objX$ is the element physical position, $kDegreesVision$ is a constant that determines the device angle of view, $kWidthPixels$ is the width of the device display, and $kXAxisRight$ and $kXAxisLeft$ define respectively the right and left flanks of the display. Depending on the user point of view ($compass$ value) the display representation is redrawn. If the object is out of field of vision, we need to decide if adjust it in the left side or in the right side. This is solved with the first condition of equation 1.

---

[2] http://www.w3.org/TR/owl-features/

3.3.2 Y-Asis (Accelereometer)

Again, we need to know if the object is inside of the angle of view. The condition is the same changing the *compass* values to accelerometer (*acclmrt*) values. When the object is inside, the equation 4 returns the position of the object in pixels. In the other hand, the condition returns whether the object is situated in the top or the lower side of the screen (equation 3)

$$pY \begin{cases} Abs(objY - acclrmtr) > \left(\dfrac{kAcclrmtrVision}{2}\right) : pY = \begin{cases} (objY - acclrmtr) > \left(\dfrac{kAcclrmtrVision}{2}\right) : pY = kYAxisUp \\ (objY - acclrmtr) <= \left(\dfrac{kAcclrmtrVision}{2}\right) : pY = kYAxisDown \end{cases} \quad (3) \\ Abs(objY - acclrmtr) <= \left(\dfrac{kAcclrmtrVision}{2}\right) : pY = (objY - acclrmtr) * \left(\dfrac{kHightPixels}{kAcclrmtrVision}\right) + \left(\dfrac{kHightPixels}{2}\right) \quad (4) \end{cases}$$

3.4 Specific Implementation

We have used the mobile device iPhone (3GS version with iOS 4.2) in our study case. This device has 320x480 pixels of screen, so its dimensions are suitable for our purpose, the mobile augmented reality. It has integrated accelerometer and digital compass sensors that we use to locate objects in vertical and horizontal axis respectively.

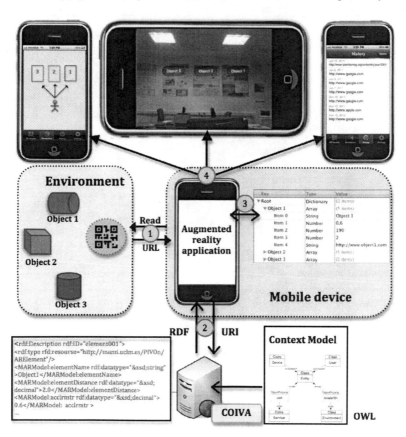

Fig. 1. General architecture of the MARM framework

In Figure 1, we show the whole process where the information is obtained from a server and is represented into the screen of the device. First, the device has to read the QR code that contains an URL. This URL corresponds to the server storing information that will be downloaded (1). In the next step, the device requests the information to the server, which will respond with the file that contains the environment representing RDF (2). After that, the application gets from a Property List[3] file the parameters that describe where is every object (3). Finally, the user has the possibility of seeing the objects in the 2D map or in the augmented reality view (4).

4 Ambient Assisted Living Applications

The MARM model and the iPhone-based implementation have been applied to actual problems of elderly people living alone. Table 1 shows several examples including the semantic rules applied to adapt the shown information and several illustrative pictures. The first example tries to help in the performance of daily activities such as

Table 1. Examples of mobile augmented-reality for Ambient Assisted Living

Application	Pictures
How to put the washer on.	
Semantics	Not applicable
How to prepare meat depending on the current medical situation, for example based on arterial pressure or glucose level.	
Semantics	Biometrical signals obtained from MoMo framework [11].
Which medicament the user has to take and when is the next doctor's appointment.	
Semantics (SWRL)	MobileDevice (?m) & User (?u) & owner (?u,?m) & medicine (?md) & swrlb:lessThan ((op:substract-dates (now (?t) & dose (?md, ?u)), doseMargin (?md)) => toShowAR (?md, ?u)

---

[3] http://developer.apple.com/library/mac/#documentation/Cocoa/
Conceptual/PropertyLists/CreatePropListProgram/CreatePropList
Program.html

putting the washer machine on or switches the heating on. The second example provides information about what meat to cook and shows the steps to perform it. In this case, the system choices among several recipes depending on the current biometrical signals of the user that can be obtained from proposals like MoMo Framework [11] and can be integrated in the context model. Finally, the third example infers the application behavior through SWRL[4] rules based on the medicaments need of the user at that moment. Also it detects when the user needs to request medicines and updates the augmented-reality-based calendar with the physician appointment.

5 Conclusions

This paper presents an infrastructure to support augmented-reality-based information adaptability for elderly or dependent users by describing context information with Semantic Web languages. A general model represents the information to show and the mechanisms to transform the physical location of objects into a mobile user interface. Also, we have presented a specific implementation using iPhone technology and making use of characteristics such as accelerometer and digital compass.

This approach allows the automatic generation of augmented-reality-based user interfaces at run-time with the necessary dynamism for adapting users' needs according to their context. This model and application is especially suitable to users than need to be guide or helped in their daily activities like occurs in typical AAL scenarios. In addition, this kind of services makes easy to relatives and assistants the supervision of what is happening at home (medicines doses, feeding, activities, etc.) and to detect incidences at the moment they occurs.

Acknowledgments. This work has been financed by the TIN2010-20510-C04-04 project from the Ministerio de Ciencia e Innovación (Spain).

References

1. European Commission. Ambient Assisted Living Joint Programme, http://www.aal-europe.eu/ (last visit January, 2011)
2. Jara, A.J., Alcazar, N., Zamora, M.A., Skarmeta, A.F.G., Istepanian, R.S.H., Sungoor, A.: Diabetes Management and Insulin Therapy in the Hospital and AAL environments based on Mobile Health. In: International Workshop on Ambient Assisted Living (IWAAL), Garceta, Madrid, pp. 7–16 (2010)
3. Bravo, J., López-de-Ipiña, D., Fuentes, C., Hervás, R., Peña, R., Vergara, M., Casero, G.: Enabling NFC technology for supporting chronic diseases: A proposal for alzheimer caregivers. In: Aarts, E., Crowley, J.L., de Ruyter, B., Gerhäuser, H., Pflaum, A., Schmidt, J., Wichert, R. (eds.) AmI 2008. LNCS, vol. 5355, pp. 109–125. Springer, Heidelberg (2008)
4. Raso, I., Hervás, R., Bravo, J.: m-Physio: Personalized Accelerometer-based Physical Rehabilitation Platform. In: Fourth International Conference on Mobile Ubiquitous Computing, Systems, Services and Technologies, IARIA (2010)

---

[4] http://www.w3.org/Submission/SWRL/

5. Vergara, M., Díaz-Hellín, P., Fontecha, J., Hervás, R., Sánchez-Barba, C., Fuentes, C., Bravo, J.: Mobile prescription: An NFC-based proposal for AAL. In: 2nd International Workshop on Near Field Communication, pp. 27–32 (2010)
6. Bravo, J., Hervás, R., Fontecha, J.: Touch-based Services' Catalogs for AAL. In: Daniel, F., Facca, F.M. (eds.) ICWE 2010. LNCS, vol. 6385, pp. 459–462. Springer, Heidelberg (2010)
7. López-de-Ipiña, D., Díaz-de-Sarralde, I., García-Zubia, J.: An ambient assisted living platform integrating RFID data-on-tag care annotations and Twitter. J. of Univer. Compu. Sci. 16(12), 1521–1538 (2010), doi:10.3217/jucs-016-12
8. Bretón-López, J., Quero, S., Botella, C., García-Palacios, A., Baños, R.M., Alcañiz, M.: An Augmented Reality System Validation for the Treatment of Cockroach Phobia. J. Cyberpsycho. Behav. 13(6), 705–710 (2010), doi:10.1089/cyber.2009.0170
9. Hervás, R., Bravo, J., Fontecha, J.: A context model based on ontological languages, a proposal for information visualization. J. Univers. Comput. Sci. 16(12), 1539–1555 (2010), doi:10.3217/jucs-016-12
10. Hervas, R., Bravo, J.: COIVA: Context-aware and Ontology-powered Information Visualization Architecture. Software Pract. Exper. (2011), doi:10.1002/spe.1011
11. Villarreal, V., Laguna, J., López, S., Fontecha, J., Fuentes, C., Hervás, R., De Ipiña, D.L., Bravo, J.: A proposal for mobile diabetes self-control: Towards a patient monitoring framework. In: Omatu, S., Rocha, M.P., Bravo, J., Fernández, F., Corchado, E., Bustillo, A., Corchado, J.M. (eds.) IWANN 2009. LNCS, vol. 5518, pp. 870–877. Springer, Heidelberg (2009)

Using and Applying MobiPattern to Design MoMo Framework Modules

Vladimir Villarreal[1], Jesus Fontecha[2], Ramon Hervás[2], and José Bravo[2]

[1] Technological University of Panama, Panama, Republic of Panama
vladimir.villarreal@utp.ac.pa
[2] MAmI Research Lab, University of Castilla-La Mancha, Ciudad Real, Spain
{jesus.fontecha,jose.bravo,ramon.hlucas}@uclm.es

Abstract. Patients constant monitoring is considered one of the most relevant aspects in healthcare. The development of a framework to communicate information between mobile and biometric devices allows constant monitoring of the patient, is viewed as a solution to healthcare issues. In this paper, we define an important element in framework design. This element we called "MobiPattern" that allow the development of standardized modules, to finally generate the final mobile monitoring application. Each module has a specific functionality and relationship with other modules. First of all, we define the characteristics of each "MobiPattern" with functional structure and finally, we evaluate the generation of each module based on a particular "MobiPattern".

Keywords: Model-driven Development, Mobile Computing, Ambient Assisted Living, Ontology, Design Patterns.

1 Introduction

Deployment patterns that allow rapid, flexible and orderly development application have great importance in the development framework structures or generation application. Actually exist some project to define and development patterns to design mobile application. In [1] they study how the design patterns can support organisational memory in mobile application design. Some studies have used patterns in different areas, facilitating the prototypes, applications and interfaces development. In [2], has developed a series of reusable, flexible itinerary patterns that enables rapid development of complex itineraries agents. It's used in conjunction with a library of tasks; these patterns of itineraries have reduced time of development agent's of forty percent. For its part [3], describes the development of to pattern language that enables the mobile in a multimodal dialogue system interaction design. The freeware on the mobile device shows the flexibility of this approach, even though not generated and graphic elements ad hoc provisions. Some research use Model-Driven Architecture (MDA) for generating code of mobile applications. In [4] the graphical models are then used to generate the corresponding XML descriptions of the mobile user interface and the workflow specification. We have developed an architecture framework that allows construction or generation of interactive applications [5] that will be embedded in the mobile device (PDA, mobile phone, etc.). This user will have

J. Bravo, R. Hervás, and V. Villarreal (Eds.): IWAAL 2011, LNCS 6693, pp. 25–32, 2011.
© Springer-Verlag Berlin Heidelberg 2011

the functionality you need to use in the program, depending on previously selected parameters. The wizard will create the source code of to complete program with such functionality. As part our research we have defined different ontologies [6] to allow the data communication between modules. This framework allows the patient multi mobile monitoring. On the other hand, [7] propose a patient Tele-monitoring process. He proposes using a monitoring device; a person (patient or assistant) should be able of just touching a NFC (*Near Field Communication*) tag with the phone, in order to launch the mobile phone application. As a result, the monitoring device should be active and the measures sent to the mobile phone through a Bluetooth connection. This application makes a recommendation through mobile phone. The use of such technologies is contemplated due to the low cost and energy consumption.

2   Functionality of Each MobiPattern and the Relationship with the Previous Defined Ontologies (Definition and Classification)

Mobile applications differ greatly from desktop applications. Users not used in the same way, do not expect the same capabilities, and in some cases are typically used in a complementary manner. They have characteristics that make it completely different from the other applications, especially in the runtime environment. Here are some situations that lead us to design and develop appropriate for these applications, depending on the functionality and requirements with which count of elements. This section discusses the generation of mobile applications for monitoring patients within a high level of abstraction. In our study we have development of specific modules with functions defined for each of the requirements that have to create an application for mobile device.

For the creation of these modules and integration of each of them for the generation of mobile applications have defined and developed a set of patterns called "**MobiPattern**", classified in the following items listed in Figure 1. For the definition of any MobiPattern we have to consider all the interpretations made are generated

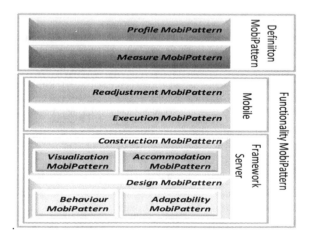

Fig. 1. Patterns used for generating application stack

after the measurement. Looking for the "multi-monitoring", all measurements made by a given biometric device reads will have five levels of ranges alert, low, acceptable, ideal and high.

In this section we will be explain the functionality of each MobiPattern structure and the relationship with specific ontology.

Definition MobiPattern: *Profile MobiPattern*

The patient profile is one of the most important element of our framework architectural elements since according to the specifications this note will be generated each modules required for viewing. The *Profile* **MobiPattern** is responsible for generating the patient profile especially associated with the disease of the patient. It's compounded by *id, name, address, phonenum, housenum, contact, email* and *disease.*

Definition MobiPattern: *Measure MobiPattern*

Besides the patient profile, it is necessary to generate a **MobiPattern** that generates a measure module. This MobiPattern have three elements as show in the upper position of figure 2b: *measurerangeH*, that define the high measure range in a measurement, *meausrerangeL* that define the low range in a measurement and level that define one level of the five level of a measure, explained in a before section. This MobiPattern undertakes to manipulate reads each of vital signs, biometric devices in such a way that the application constantly monitors the patient and know-generated in due course modules in the application *launch* when needed.

Functionality MobiPattern: *Design MobiPattern*

Its enables us to define the structures of our application functionality, as the application will be executed on the mobile device. Taking into account that although the technical performance of our mobile phone is powerful enough as to process large amounts of information, not comparable to benefits that provide a conventional computer. That is why generated applications must able to conform to the size of each device on which to run. In this regard are defined two **MobiPattern** essential at the time of building applications for mobile devices based on aspects of functionality and adaptability.

Functionality MobiPattern: *Design MobiPattern - Behavior MobiPttern*

This **MobiPattern** defines the various features of each module. Here is where it is established that parameters are required for a module, which are processes that are running and what the end of each output, as show in figure 2a. That is ***what makes each module?***

Functionality MobiPattern: *Design MobiPattern* - **Adaptability MobiPattern**

This MobiPattern defines the possibility to adapt news capabilities to applications, for interact with existing ones. That is ***how integrates a new module functionality?*** or ***How to create a new module from existing ones***? This **MobiPattern** functionality includes the following case show in figure 2b: there are two modules previously created through its behavior **MobiPattern** and have the need to create a new module that has a new functionality that uses features of these two previous modules. Applying adaptability **MobiPattern**, adjust these values to build a new module with a new behavior **MobiPattern**. When you need the same module again won't need adapting because it has been created for that patient.

Functionality MobiPattern: Construction MobiPattern

Construction **MobiPattern** define the way in which after designed modules will be integrated in a single application to be executed on the mobile device. It must take into account that generated applications that will be embedded in the mobile phone must have functionality delimited each patient so not loaded items that will not be used. With these **MobiPattern** location or accommodation of each module in the application are defined and it chosen and configured all display parameters thus adapted to the mobile device that will be used.

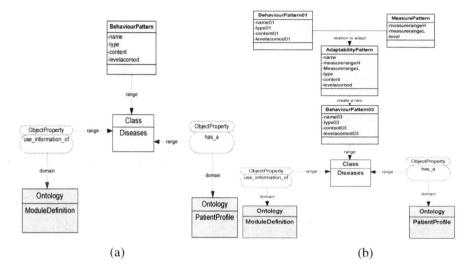

(a)   (b)

Fig. 2. a. Behavior MobiPattern for each condition and its relationship with the ontology structure. b. Structure of Adaptability MobiPattern to every disease.

Functionality MobiPattern: Construction MobiPattern - *Accommodation MobiPattern*

It defines the location of each module or element in the application structure. You must view onto one screen different functionalities for a patient without the need of having to surf much application. We have been defined level to location elements, with the function of each of these levels. In fact, ***where to locate each element?*** For easier handling and construction of this **MobiPattern**, we have defined three levels of accommodation when building applications: ***Bottom level or adjustments (Low Level)*** here are all the modules for adjustments or changes to make to the application so that if the vital signs readings vary much this level should know to communicate this need to the time that is required. Here is located also predictive model that receives constant information at the time of reading changes in vital signs received biometric device in periods of time, ***Level medium or control (Average Level)*** here are all the other modules that correspond to the monitoring of the patient, i.e. if a patient suffers from a certain disease, at this level only have modules to help you manage this disease and ***Top level or measurement (Top Level)*** the highest level in the accommodation MobiPattern, in this one, the application runs with higher priority reading and constant interpretation of changes in a patient's vital signs informing layers more inferior must be running at the time that is required.

When developing applications we long term this pattern to locate three levels corresponding to each application modules. This is done with the objective prioritization of location on the device for later use in the execution MobiPattern.

Functionality MobiPattern: Construction MobiPattern - *Visualization MobiPattern* It defines the visual parameters of the application at the time of being generated for the various types of mobile devices. Items evaluated are dimension, resolution and type of device, among others. These three elements must be adapted to be visible on any device: hardware, software and communication specifications. That is *what output format is most appropriate?* This MobiPattern is related to the mobile devices that we defined in the previous section so that you need to know all types, brands, models and specifications of each device to thus adapt the output adjusted to technical requirements of each user.

Functionality MobiPattern: Execution MobiPattern

This **MobiPattern** is helpful, allowing you to define which elements are related to each other after generated application for mobile device. You must define which modules are considered for analysis, which for processing and which to display information. Here is where is located the features previously designed by **MobiPattern** behavior. That is *what elements run to monitor the patient?*. Defined here **MobiPattern** to generate subsistence, self-control, suggestions, recommendations, alerts, etc.

Functionality MobiPattern: Readjustment MobiPattern

After generated application monitoring for a patient, and taking into account potential variations or significant deterioration of a patient's vital signs, framework must be able to redefine or readjust the application previously generated in the mobile device. That is *what change or update?* and *when to do it?* **MobiPattern** adjustment has the function of generating modules changes or adjustments to the application previously generated for the mobile device, so that if you need to make changes to the original application, it knows where to make these changes. Mentioning this last, the changes you can make the entire application, generating again or certain modules, updating them on the mobile device. This adjustment can be done in two specific times, either an extremely urgent alert will be generated and prompted immediate readjustment or changes are not of much importance level and you can expect the next visit to the doctor. In both cases the monitoring application, stores any need to change or adjustment to be made. Then framework check if some readjustment querying application module was generated, and it automatically communicates whether needed or not (**needchange**, *true* or *false*) and make the appropriate updates (**namemodule**). When all the necessary elements has been updated, is to update the application or modules previously generated in the mobile device.

3   Generating Modules Based on the MobiPatterns

We will evaluate the functionality of the definition of a MobiPattern for the generation of applications that facilitates the monitoring of patients. This set an activity flow that will continue to facilitate the understanding of the process of generation of modules for control of patients.

a. Visit to the medical doctor/specialist: we began with a medical consultation made a patient suffering from diabetes. The patient arrives at their medical consultation with your doctor; the patient has a glucometer units glucose and in addition a mobile control. It is your first consultation therefore patient reported discomfort that has, the doctor makes relevant exams diagnosing diabetes.

b. Creation and updating of the patient profile (MobiPattern Profile evaluation) Patient Profile update: what makes Dr. initially create the patient profile, is treat you the application on your personal computer, which starts the registration data of the patient, on the basis of the information being queried and we have defined in the generated ontologies, which facilitate the Organization and analysis of information that the patient has.

c. Creation and updating of modules (each MobiPattern evaluation): it is this section comes to the creation of the modules that are involved in the generation of schemas for each of the MobiPattern-based applications. Specific modules based on your profile and the type of disease that suffers are created for each type of patient.

d. Creation and updating of the Measure module (Measure MobiPattern): one of the most important modules is module measures, through critical signals generated by the biometric device values are obtained, and define module must be running on the application of monitoring. As this pattern is related to the type of disease, there may be a measure for each type of vital signal, i.e. one to measure blood glucose others to measure voltage, another for measuring temperature and run modules for each of them or otherwise measures relate to run modules common module. In figure 3a shows the functionality of this pattern to the patient that we are evaluating. After generated module measures and created each of the modules, the application displays the patient some options depending on the level obtained by the reading of its vital signal, i.e. depending on the measurement result, appears the patient choices he chooses.

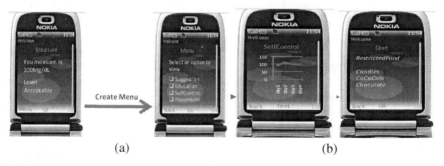

(a)   (b)

Fig. 3. a. Menu for patient monitoring applications generation. b. MobiPattern BehaviourPattern for the generation of: a."Self-Control" module seen graphically user evaluation, b.Diet.

e. Creation and updating of the modules: Education, Suggestion, Prevention, Self-Control, Diet and Alert (Behaviour MobiPattern evaluation): these modules are considered functional, because they are the basis of the relationship profile - measure. Information that shows each module is part of each of the ontologies that have been described previously, and which acquires the values needed for each patient. Each of the generated modules have interpretation (normal, ideal, low and high type) ranks every measure of the patient, by which each module is associated to a specific State of the moment in which the patient has taken such action. This is why functional modules will change according to the physical situation of the patient as show in figure 3b.

f. Creation and updating of the adaptability modules (MobiPattern Adaptability Pattern evaluation): in figure 4a we see the general and functional schema MobiPattern adaptability (AdaptabilityPattern) and the relationship between each of its elements. To create a new module with features similar to other modules, or to modify the functionality of the module created previously, there is a relationship between that previously created module and the module of measure, which collects information and adapting this new functionality into a new module. In figure 4b, show how this MobiPattern linking module Suggestion with the steps to generate a new module NewSuggestion, as it was requested that adaptation to the new module in any part of the application schema.

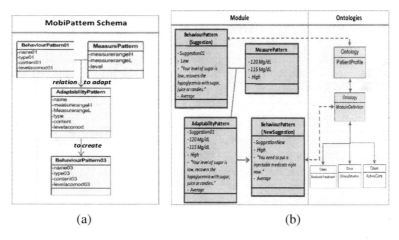

(a)   (b)

Fig. 4. Evaluation of MobiPattern AdaptabilityPattern for the generation of a new module a. master view, b. module view

g. Accommodation modules for the generation of applications. (MobiPattern AcommodationPattern evaluation): how to locate each of the modules generated for our application is one of the main functions of the accommodation MobiPattern (AccommodationPattern). This MobiPattern is responsible for defining three levels (top, average and low) location for each of its elements. These three levels define the priority that should run each of the modules. The MobiPattern definition (Profile MobiPattern and Measure MobiPattern) running in the foreground and occupy the "*Top Level*" of the accommodation MobiPattern. Similarly all functionality MobiPattern (Suggestion, Prevention, Alert, Diet, among other) run in the background, in the "*Average Level*". In the lowest level runs the predictive model and adjustment of application modules. This MobiPattern provides the location of each elements in the generation of the final application.

h. Specification of the characteristic of readjustment modules: the framework generates a module adjustment that stores the list of modules that need to be re-adjusted when running this monitoring application. This adjustment can be evaluated on the next visit to the doctor or can be generated through an alert emergency where required be changed immediately. Once generated each module, create a final application is embedded in the mobile device of the patient, which is synchronized with the biometric device.

4 Conclusions

The most important element of the framework development is the appropriate definition of MobiPattern and the relationship of each ontologies defined in a previous papers. This structure of MobiPattern allows the creation and updated of different modules for the generation of final application. Doctors have a server application when they have all information about the patient profile and the relationship with a specific disease, based in control elements, like diet, suggestions, recommendation, self-control, and other. Patient´s mobile phone is updated for the server application, in a first visit. These updates generate an application that allows the patient's mobile monitoring based in previous generated modules using a MobiPattern structure. The application will be update when the patient shows variations in the measure or status of disease; this is the functionality of our framework. We are developing a monitoring framework to facilitate moving the patient, using the existing communication both medical devices such as biometric devices. MoMo framework facilitates this task between the patient, medical specialists and doctors.

References

1. Ahlgren, R., Markkula, J.: Design Patterns and Organisational Memory in Mobile Application Development. In: Bomarius, F., Komi-Sirviö, S. (eds.) PROFES 2005. LNCS, vol. 3547, pp. 143–156. Springer, Heidelberg (2005)
2. Daria, C.N., et al.: Rapid application development using agent itinerary patterns (2000)
3. Sonntag, D.: Interaction design and implementation for multimodal mobile semantic web interfaces. In: Smith, M.J., Salvendy, G. (eds.) HCII 2007. LNCS, vol. 4558, pp. 645–654. Springer, Heidelberg (2007)
4. Abramowicz, W., Dunkel, J., Bruns, R.: Model-driven architecture for mobile applications. In: Abramowicz, W. (ed.) BIS 2007. LNCS, vol. 4439, pp. 464–477. Springer, Heidelberg (2007)
5. Villarreal, V., Laguna, J., López, S., Fontecha, J., Fuentes, C., Hervás, R., de Ipiña, D.L., Bravo, J.: A Proposal for Mobile Diabetes Self-control: Towards a Patient Monitoring Framework. In: Omatu, S., Rocha, M.P., Bravo, J., Fernández, F., Corchado, E., Bustillo, A., Corchado, J.M. (eds.) IWANN 2009. LNCS, vol. 5518, pp. 870–877. Springer, Heidelberg (2009)
6. Villarreal, V., et al.: Applying ontologies in the development of patient mobile monitoring framework. In: 2nd International Conference on e-Health and Bioengineering - EHB 2009. IEEE, Constata (2009)
7. Bravo, J., López-de-Ipiña, D., Fuentes, C., Hervás, R., Peña, R., Vergara, M., Casero, G.: Enabling NFC technology for supporting chronic diseases: A proposal for alzheimer caregivers. In: Aarts, E., Crowley, J.L., de Ruyter, B., Gerhäuser, H., Pflaum, A., Schmidt, J., Wichert, R., et al. (eds.) AmI 2008. LNCS, vol. 5355, pp. 109–125. Springer, Heidelberg (2008)

Indoor Navigation and Product Recognition for Blind People Assisted Shopping

Diego López-de-Ipiña, Tania Lorido, and Unai López

Deusto Institute of Technology – DeustoTech., University of Deusto
Avda. Universidades 24, 48007 Bilbao, Spain
{dipina,tania.lorido,unai.lopez}@deusto.es

Abstract. Achieving blind people autonomous shopping in a supermarket is a real challenge. Without help from another person is very hard or impossible for them to reach to a specific supermarket section and browse through its products. Besides, once there, they cannot identify the products and their features (e.g. price, brand and due date) to decide whether they want to buy them or not. This work presents BlindShopping, an RFID and QR-code based mobile solution to enable accessible shopping for blind people, only demanding inexpensive off-the-shelf technology and limiting the deployment effort from the supermarket.

Keywords: Blind, Navigation, Mobile Computing, QR codes, Web-Services.

1 Introduction

Although technology seems to be invading every aspect of our lives, it is still having limited impact on those social collectives which most need it, i.e. dependable people due to sensorial impairments or advanced age. Ambient Assisted Living (AAL) aims to address this gap by using ICT technology to enhance the daily activities of dependable people, e.g. blind or deaf people.

The PIRAmIDE project[1] aims to approach the AAL vision by exploiting smartphones' potential –mobile phones equipped with continuously increasing computing, communication and sensing capabilities– as sensorial complements for disabled users'. It enables the smartphone-mediated interaction of a user with the ecosystem of services populating an environment (e.g. home or supermarket). Thus, it allows disabled people to perform daily life tasks autonomously and independently of their disability (e.g. blind, deaf or elderly people). In essence, through PIRAmIDE, mobile devices are transformed into sense enhancers giving a 6th sense to those who already enjoy their five functional senses, but more importantly, complementing those which have some sensorial impairment.

One of the concrete application domains targeted by PIRAmIDE is overcoming the difficulties blind people usually encounter whilst they are shopping autonomously, as if they could see, without the help of someone else. The focus of this work is to describe an inexpensive easily-deployable solution addressing this issue, entirely based on off-the-shelf technology (mainly smartphones).

Comparative studies [3] on research for blind people assisted shopping support consider that an ideal assistive infrastructure should address the following functional and non-functional design requirements:

J. Bravo, R. Hervás, and V. Villarreal (Eds.): IWAAL 2011, LNCS 6693, pp. 33–40, 2011.
© Springer-Verlag Berlin Heidelberg 2011

- *Eyes-free product selection and browsing.* The capability of allowing blind people to easily select or browse through the available range of products, just before she initiates her purchasing process. The idea is to give blind people the chance to easily plan their shopping by knowing and selecting what products are on offer.

- *Free navigating within the store.* Once a blind person has prepared a shopping list (*planned shopping*) or rather prefers to go to different supermarket sections to browse and choose products (*opportunistic shopping*), the blind person must be offered support to navigate through the supermarket and reach to the wished section.

- *Product search and navigation.* Once the user is in the area where a product category is located, the blind person must be able of locating the concrete products types of her interest, and select the actual units she wants to purchase.

- *Utilization of existing devices.* A blind person carries with her a white cane and a mobile phone. Therefore, if any, those are the elements that may be modified or enhanced in order to allow a blind person to safely and effectively carry out her shopping. Only inexpensive off-the-shelf already known technology by the blind should be considered to ensure acceptability.

- *Minimal environment adjustments.* Supermarkets are reluctant to introduce complex changes in their internal information management systems. Furthermore, only simple low-cost easily maintainable physical instrumentation of their premises including aisles and shelves is acceptable. Any feasible solution should leave products as they are, i.e. it must be able of recognizing and deal with standard UPC barcodes utilized in worldwide retail. Hence, it is a must that accessible shopping systems operate in real supermarkets with all their restrictions.

Our proposal, namely BlindShopping, addresses the above mentioned requirements to provide an inexpensive and feasible solution in order to ensure wide deployment from blind people and supermarket organisations. A remarkable feature of our solution is that blind people will follow the conventional shopping behaviour somebody without visual problems follows.

2   Related Work

Robocart [4], developed by Utah State University, gave place to a robotic supermarket assistant, in the form of a custom-built market cart equipped with a laptop, a laser range finder, and an RFID reader. For navigation, it uses the RFID reader attached to the cart and passive RFID tags scattered at different points in a supermarket. Furthermore, a wireless barcode scanner is used for product search and identification. The biggest drawback of this system, in contrast with BlindShopping, is its use of additional non-conventional costly and complex to manage devices.

The same research group developed ShopTalk [5], an alternative more wearable solution. In this case, it requires that the user carries a barcode scanner and a Ultra-Mobile Personal Computer (UMPC) in a backpack. A barcode scanner aided with two plastic stabilisers to enhance usability is used to read MSI barcodes placed in product shelves. Verbal route instructions were issued through a headphone connected to the UMPC at the blind person's backpack. Although the supermarket does not need to install and maintain any hardware, the system requires access to the supermarket's inventory control system. In contrast, BlindShopping only requires blind users to carry a lightweight smartphone equipped with a camera to read QR [2] codes attached to product shelves and to navigate through the supermarket with the aid of a white cane augmented with an RFID reader at its tip.

Another interesting assisted shopping solution is GroZi[6], which focuses on using computer vision software for detecting products. Visually-impaired people use a hand glove with a small camera and vibrating motors that provide haptic feedback. A small wearable device carries out image processing and generates haptic feedback in the two dimensional plane of the shelf for product localization and verbal feedback for identified product description. Again, BlindShopping is more easily deployable, economically and technically, since it uses a "common" device such as a smartphone and the standard white cane used for guidance.

Tinetra[7] presented at Carnegie Mellon University, offers the possibility of detecting products via a barcode or RFID reader, and then it obtains related information via GPRS from the server. However, it does not include a guiding system as BlindShopping. Interestingly, the system advocates, as in BlindShopping case, a mobile platform for accessible blind shopping. It handles both barcodes and RFID tags. Similarly to us they use a Baracode Pencil2 and a Baracoda IDBlue to scan barcodes and RFID tags, respectively.

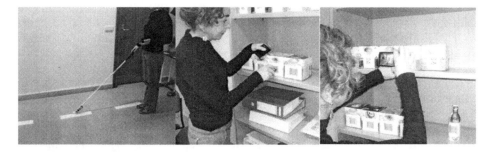

Fig. 1. Navigation system (left), UPC code recognition (middle) and QR-code recognition

iCare[8] relies on an RFID[9] reader embedded in a hand glove to detect products and query information from a server via Wi-Fi. The user has to move her hand along the shelf, so the system gives indications such as "passing dairy section". This system seems more intrusive than ours, where the user still uses her white cane, enhanced with an RFID reader. The usage of RFID is very promising, but it presents problems from the technical and industrial side. Tags attached to liquid low-end products with metal cases refract and reflect RF waves. Manufacturing costs for tags and readers remain prohibitive for tagging all but high-value products. Technical problems, environmental hazards and consumer perceptions of trust, privacy and risk, mixed with fear remain significant acceptance barriers to RFID item-level tagging.

3   The BlindShopping Platform

Our solution aims to offer eyes-free technological support for blind people to shop around as if they saw, without altering conventional shopping patterns. It is designed to avoid overloading the visually-impaired person with additional new gadgets and enforcing a supermarket to go through heavy and costly, both in price and time, installation and maintenance processes.

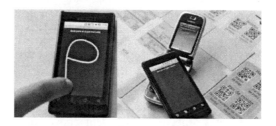

Fig. 2. User drawing a "P" (left) on Motorola Milestone, Nokia 6131 NFC to read HF RFID tag for navigation and supermarket mock-up for testing (right)

The assumptions taken by BlindShopping regarding a supermarket organization are as follows. First, it is considered that all products are grouped into different product categories (e.g. drinks), and these are divided into product types (e.g. drinks/cola) which again are divided into concrete brand products (e.g. Pepsi can). Apart from that, the supermarket area is divided into cells of two main types: cells containing a shelf and passageway cells. Thus, internally, BlindShopping maps the IDs of the RFID tags within a cell to navigation and product location information such as the type of a given cell, its neighbour cell types, and in case of being shelf type cells, the product category, types and concrete products located in that area.

BlindShopping offers infrastructural support for the whole purchasing process within a supermarket, which we understand as a four-step cyclic process: *1—product category navigation/2—product search/3—product identification/4—product selection*. Such cycle stops when the user decides to go to the cash till to pay for her purchases. Consequently, BlindShopping offers a *navigation* component driving the user through voice messages to the aisle where a product category previously dictated to her smartphone is located. Once there, BlindShopping also offers support for *product recognition* by either shelf section identification or product own identification by means of embossed QR and UPC scanning, respectively. Note that QR codes redundant encoding allows for efficient recognition even when a blind person slowly passes her mobile camera over the embossment where the code is.

Besides, BlindShopping does not only offer a working technical solution for assisted shopping, but it provides an affordable, usable and easily-manageable solution for blind people. *Affordable* since the cost of the platform deployment is relatively reduced. The supermarket must install a server and a wireless network (Wi-Fi) in the shopping area. In addition to this, RFID tags must be distributed throughout the floor (see left hand side of Fig. 1). On the other hand, the visually impaired customer must carry a smartphone, a very common device nowadays. The most significant investment would be the acquisition of RFID readers attachable to blind people's white canes bought by the supermarket and lent to its clients.

Usable since the application is adapted in a way that blind people can make an independent use of it. It includes a gesture and voice-based interface, which allows selecting among the different functionalities by drawing strokes on the smartphone screen with a finger or issuing voice commands (see Fig. 2). The rest of the interaction is done through speech synthesis and recognition. The blind user says the supermarket section where she wants to go, and the system uses speech synthesis to give routing indications or product information. Once the user is located in front of product type section (e.g. daily product/milk), she can locate specific products by pointing her phone camera in the direction where an easily recognizable embossed 2-D code (e.g. Carrefour's semi-skimmed milk) has been stuck on a shelf. Those codes are stuck on the typical plastic tags including name and price for each product distributed through the shelves of a supermarket.

Easily-manageable since the BlindShopping navigation and product type management web-based client (see Fig. 3) offers an intuitive interface to configure the RFID-tag based navigation system and the QR codes assigned to product types attached in front of the shelf portion where those products are located.

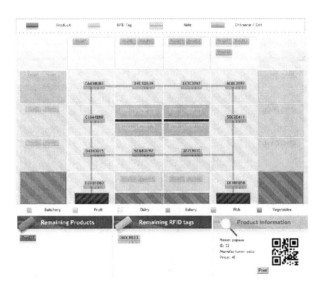

Fig. 3. BlindShopping Management Tool

4   BlindShopping Architecture

Fig. 4 shows the distributed component architecture of our solution, composed of the following three components:

1. *Navigation system.* It is in charge of guiding the blind user inside the supermarket, by giving her, through a headphone connected to her smartphone, simple verbal navigation instructions. Such component combines a white cane with a portable RFID reader attached to its tip, a set of road mark-like RFID tag lines distributed throughout the corridors of the supermarket (see left hand side of Fig. 1 and top part of Fig. 5, respectively) and a smartphone application

processing the RFID readings received though Bluetooth and generating user navigation verbal commands as result.

2. *Product recognition*. Once the user reaches the target product section, she fetches some of the products there, see Fig. 1, or better points with her camera phone to an embossed QR or UPC code attached to every section of a shelf where a different type of product has been placed. The smartphone camera recognizes that code and then informs verbally about the product main features. Note that a QR code can encode up-to 4296 alphanumeric characters, and its redundancy makes successful reading possible even when partial images of them are captured. Details about the recognized products may be encoded in the codes themselves or retrieved from the back-end.

3. *System management*: BlindShopping includes a web front-end for BlindShopping RFID and QR code infrastructure management. It allows the registration of the collection of RFID tags scattered though the supermarket floor and the QR-codes attached to shelf sections. For that, it offers a RIA (Rich Internet Application) interface which is very usable from any web browser without requiring specific technical knowledge (see Fig. 3 for more details).

4.1 Implementation and Usability Issues

A Nokia 6131 NFC has been used for reading RFID tag floor markings. A Java ME application has been developed which continuously reads RFID tags and sends their codes through Bluetooth to a mobile Android application (see Fig. 4). An easier, lighter, cheaper and more robust solution can be achieved by attaching a portable RFID reader such as a Baracoda Tagrunner[1] to the tip of the white cane. In fact, we have already created a version of the system which operates with Baracoda's ID Blue device (see centre of Fig. 5) – a more old-fashioned device with the important drawback of demanding a button press every time an RFID tag wants to be read.

The selected Android devices for our tests were a Motorola Milestone with Android 2.1 OS and an HTC Desire device with Android 2.2. With them, a blind person chooses an action by means of a gesture or by issuing a voice command. Concretely, the navigation system operation is requested by drawing an "L" or issuing the "Location" voice command (see Fig. 2). This launches the supermarket navigation system, which initially asks the user to touch a floor RFID marking or the QR code attached to a nearby product shelf to figure out where the user currently is. Next, the application requests the user to dictate the product category or type where she wants to go. Note that the smartphone maintains a Bluetooth connection with the RFID reader to keep track of where the user is at every time. As the visually impaired walks on, the android application will give verbal navigation indications ("go straight on", "turn left", "turn around" and so forth) until the target section is reached. Observe that whenever the blind person follows a wrong route, the system automatically detects it since the blind person keeps touching the floor RFID markers as she moves. Both product information and the route to be followed are obtained from the server by invoking web services accessible through a Wi-Fi connection.

Drawing a "P" or issuing a "Product" voice command, the user accesses the product recognition component that allows obtaining information about a product.

---

[1] http://www.baracoda.com/baracoda/product/p_48_TagRunners.html

The system then asks the user to point the smartphone to the shelves, so that the camera will recognize an easily detected by the blind person embossed QR or embossed UPC code (see middle and right hand side of Fig. 1) and obtain either the product details directly or the ID of the product from which its details can be retrieved from the BlindShopping back-end. By using speech synthesis, the application informs the user about the product details, e.g. its name, manufacturer and price.

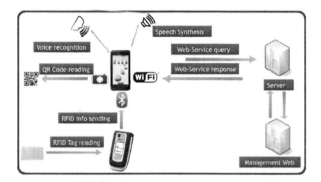

Fig. 4. BlindShopping Distributed Architecture

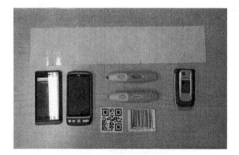

Fig. 5. RFID tag marking (top), Motorola Milestone and HTC Desire Android devices (left), Baracoda's Pencil2 barcode recognizer and IDBlue RFID reader (middle), NFC 6131 NFC device (right) and QR-Code and standard UPC barcode (bottom centre)

5   Usability Study

A basic usability study with a blind person was conducted in order to validate the usability and accessibility features of our navigation and product identification subsystems. The blind person was requested to navigate through different sections of our emulated supermarket surface by using her white cane with an attached BT RFID reader and an Android application on an HTC Desire (see Fig. 1, left hand side). Her main comment was that navigation was very intuitive since locating the RFID tag markings was very easy due to their different texture and small relief, and the navigation vocal commands were very useful to reach the desired target.

The blind person was requested to assess whether locating embossed UPC barcodes through a Baracoda Pencil2 (see centre of Fig. 1) was easier or harder than using the Android phone camera to point to embossed QR codes (see right hand side of Fig. 1). After 10 product recognitions with each alternative, she judged that the second approach was much simpler. Besides, QR code recognition using a camera phone was found to be much faster and reliable. The redundant encoding of information on embossed (easily found by touch) QR-codes allows their identification even when only a partial image of them is captured.

6 Conclusions and Further Work

This work has shown a low-cost easily deployable solution for blind people assisted shopping constituted of two main components: a) an RFID and mobile phone based indoor *navigation system* and b) a mobile QR-code based *product recognizer*. It is important to note that although the chosen scenario was a supermarket, the platform can be easily adapted to any other self-service shopping scenario.

Further work will expand the BlindShopping Android mobile application with GPS reading capabilities, so as to guide the user from her home to the supermarket. Although the RFID reader has been implemented with a Nokia NFC as a proof of concept, it will soon be replaced by a dedicated Bluetooth RFID reader. A fully fledge evaluation in a real supermarket carried out by a statistically significant group of blind people will also be carried out to thoroughly assess the suitability of the proposed solution.

The prototyped solution can be seen online at Youtube[8]. This work has been supported by project grant TSI-020301-2008-2 (PIRAmIDE), funded by the Spanish Ministry of Industry, Tourism and Commerce. We want to thank Mercedes Mata for evaluating the system.

References

1. PIRAmIDE platform official site (2011), http://www.piramidepse.com
2. QR Code ISO specification (2011), http://tinyurl.com/4dnub9e
3. Kulyukin, V., Kutiyanawala, A.: Accessible Shopping Systems for Blind and Visually Impaired Individuals: Design Requirements and the State of the Art. The Open Rehabilitation Journal 3, 158–168 (2010)
4. Kulyukin, V., Gharpure, C., Nicholson, J.: RoboCart: Toward robot-assisted navigation of grocery stores by the visually impaired. In: Proceedings of the IEEE/RSJ IROS, pp. 2845–2850. IEEE Press, Edmonton (2005)
5. Nicholson, J., Kulyukin, V.: ShopTalk: Independent blind shopping = verbal route directions + barcode scans. In: Proceedings of the 30th Rehabilitation Engineering and Assistive Technology Society of North America (RESNA), Phoenix, USA (2007)
6. Merler, M., Galleguillos, C., Belongie, S.: Recognizing groceries in situ using in vitro training data. SLAM, Minneapolis (2007)
7. Lanigan, P.E., Paulos, A.M., Williams, A.W., Rossi, D., Narasimhan, P.: Trinetra: Assistive technologies for grocery shopping for the blind. In: International IEEE-BAIS Symposium on Research on Assistive Technologies (RAT). Dayton, OH (2007)
8. Project demonstration, Youtube (2011),
   http://www.youtube.com/watch?v=XS53XjSihQQ
9. Krishna, S., Balasubramanian, V., Krishnan, N.C., Hedgpeth, T.: The iCARE Ambient interactive shopping environment. In: 23rd Annual International Technology and Persons with Disabilities Conference (CSUN), Los Angeles, CA (2008)

Easing the Mobility of Disabled People in Supermarkets Using a Distributed Solution

Aitor Gómez-Goiri[1], Eduardo Castillejo[1], Pablo Orduña[1], Xabier Laiseca[1],
Diego López-de-Ipiña[1], and Sergio Fínez[2]

[1] Deusto Institute of Technology - DeustoTech
University of Deusto
Avda. Universidades 24, 48007 Bilbao, Spain
{aitor.gomez,eduardo.castillejo,pablo.orduna,
xabier.laiseca,dipina}@deusto.es
http://www.morelab.deusto.es
[2] Treelogic
Parque Tecnológico de Asturias Parcela 30
Llanera, E33428 Asturias, Spain
sergio.finez@treelogic.com
http://www.treelogic.com

Abstract. People's impairments cause a wide range of difficulties in
everyday tasks. Particularly, handicapped people face many challenges
both at home, but especially outside it, where their reduced mobility is a
burden. Buying in a supermarket can be sometimes troublesome for them
and so as to facilitate this task, a product locator application is proposed.
This application runs on heterogeneous personal mobile devices keeping
the user private information safe on them, and it locates the desired
products over each supermarket's map.

Keywords: shopping, mobility, disability, mobile devices, triple space.

1 Introduction

Some of the most common impairments that disabled people suffer are some-
how related to mobility. Indeed, impairments not directly related to mobility
can easily derive in causing disabled people to move slowly in a normal environment. These mobility limitations often become worse in crowded places such as
supermarkets, where avoiding people and remembering where to go depending
on the desired products becomes challenging. Applications specifically designed
to enhance the shopping experience, i.e. guide applications, can easily palliate
these difficulties.

The solution proposed in this paper displays products' location over a supermarket map, so disabled customers can decide the better route. Its data is
fully distributed on their mobile devices and in the supermarket servers where
common information is held. This approach is respectful with the privacy of the
users, but yet lets them locate where they must go next inside the supermarket.

J. Bravo, R. Hervás, and V. Villarreal (Eds.): IWAAL 2011, LNCS 6693, pp. 41–48, 2011.

Although this application will be useful for any kind of customer, people with mobility limitations will benefit most as the time they spend moving when they are buying will be considerably reduced. Doing so, the stress that such kind of crowded places generates in them is expected to be palliated, resulting in a better shopping experience.

The remainder of the paper is organized as follows. Section 2 discusses related work. Section 3 presents a use case where the solution will be used. Section 4 details the technical aspects of the proposed solution. Finally, Section 5 concludes and outlines the future work.

2   Related Work

With ageing of Europe [8], the infrastructures used for treating the elderly will gain relevance, and the costs of these infrastructures will increase notably. In order to optimize the costs of these infrastructures, the development of new technical solutions is required. Given that the ageing of the population causes physical disabilities, it is expected that the number of users with physical disabilities will increase in the near future. The elderly of the population is a problem that the European Union is addressing by the promotion of programmes to develop applications and frameworks that enable the reduction of related costs and the increasing of factors that ease the quality of elderly's life. Within this context, Ambient Assisted Living [2] solutions are arising across Europe to tackle these costs.

Efforts are being placed in supporting an automatic system that guides disabled users in a known system, as reported in [7]. However, these systems require that the supermarket provides an indoor location system, which is not the case in the supermarkets we work with. Therefore, no automatic guiding algorithm can be implemented within the supermarket.

The use case presented in this paper is formed by several independent nodes which share their information. In order to share it in a very decoupled but expressive way TS paradigm [3] is used. TS comes from tuplespace-based coordination languages where the interaction between processes is performed sharing information in a common space. Although, several approaches in the field of semantic tuplespaces exist [6,5], to the best of our knowledge this kind of solution has never been specifically designed and implemented to use mobile devices as another peer of these semantic spaces and not only as simple clients apart from in our middleware [4].

3   Use Case Description

The target of the developed platform is to enable elderly and disabled people to optimize the search of products in supermarkets. We expect that for certain types of disabilities, such as physical disabilities that make them move slowly in a supermarket -requiring wheelchairs, or just walking slowly-, will be more willing to go to supermarkets if their shopping experience is considerably better, by finding the desired products immediately.

In order to achieve this, users will first use a mobile application in their mobile device, technically described in section 4.1, on which they will select which products will try to buy in the supermarket. They will be able to do this task wherever they are: at home, work, in the street... The mobile application will connect to the supermarkets global servers through the TS and it will retrieve which products are available, and at what price. In this first application version, we do not include more information, although supermarkets usually have other information such as products preview images that would increase the shopping experience. For instance, ALIMERKA[1] lists the available products, prices, codes and images. Once products are listed in the mobile application, users will select from the list what items are willing to buy.

Then, at some point of the week, users go to the supermarket. They will be able to ask for a device with the *product locator application* (technically described in 4.2) already deployed. These devices will typically be tablets such as Apple iPad or Samsung Galaxy Tab, properly tagged so users can't leave the supermarket with them. In fact, similar technologies are already provided to users in a secure way in restaurants [1] to let users select the products, pay and even play videogames.

Once they have the device, users will launch the *shopping cart application* in their own mobile device. Then, users will write their username in the *shopping cart application*, which automatically will retrieve the selected products from the users' mobile devices. With this information, the *product locator application* will query to a server placed in the supermarket for the location and availability of the selected products and it will show in a seamless way those available products in a map of the supermarket. With this information, users can go through the supermarket with the customized map in their hands.

This solution is built within the ACROSS project[2] (TSI-020301-2009-27), funded by the Spanish Ministerio de Industria, Turismo y Comercio. The project aims to build social robotics services in certain areas, including supermarkets. Therefore, it is expected that in the near future the *product locator application* will run on the TICO robot, developed by Treelogic and Adele Robots[3].

The robot will then guide users if there are not many users waiting for the robot and if there is enough battery left. Otherwise the map of the *product locator application* might be showed or the system would rely on the tablet acquisition by users or the automatic deployment of the *product locator application* in the user's mobile phone. Within the project, this system is expected to be deployed in certain ALIMERKA supermarkets in Spain. Since a network infrastructure and the maintenance costs are assumed by the supermarket, the system can't be deployed in every supermarket.

---

[1] www.alimerka.es

[2] www.acrosspse.com

[3] www.adelerobots.com

4   System Architecture

The system is divided into three main elements (see Fig. 1), the mobile Shopping Cart application allows users to search for supermarket products; the Products Manager, which main purpose is to manage each supermarket product list (e.g. adding another milk brand); and the Product Locator application, which finds and locates in the different supermarket's corridors and shelves where users' desired products are.

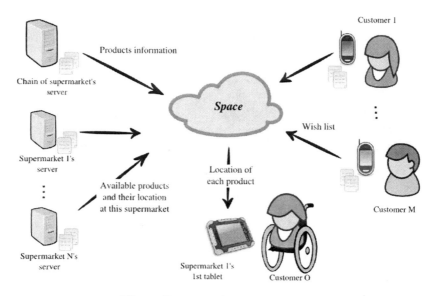

Fig. 1. System architecture diagram

These applications share information between them using a common space where they can write and also make queries as shown in 1.

4.1   Shopping Cart Mobile Application

In order to encourage the users to note down the products they are willing to buy, a "todo list"-like Android[4] application has been designed to be run on the user's personal mobile phone. Doing so, the user can benefit from our solution not only being guided in the supermarket, but also avoiding inconvenient oversights.

The proposed *shopping cart application* connects to different triple spaces. First, the user must identify himself in the application (see Fig. 2a), then to retrieve the list of all available products in a chain of supermarkets the global space is used (see Fig. 2b). Finally he connects to a users' space, where the concrete shopping list of each user (see Fig. 2c) is written. Due to the implementation of the used TS solution, the data written by the user in his mobile phone will stay

---

[4] www.android.com

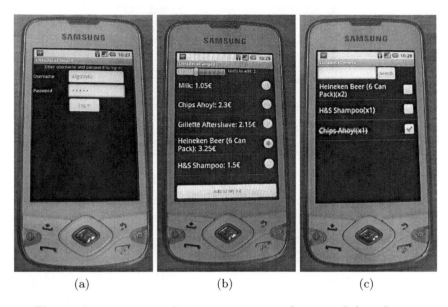

Fig. 2. *shopping cart application* running on a Samsung Galaxy Spyca

at his device considering privacy issues but it will be accessible by the *product locator application* whenever the mobile is connected to the space.

4.2 Product Locator Tablet Application

Trying to find out where our shopping list products are in a supermarket can be tedious and ponderous. Supermarkets tend to change products shelves, bringing new market brands and putting special offers in the end podium every month.

The presented Android application focuses on helping users with this task. By querying Ts, wish list's products will be drawn over the current supermarket map (see Fig. 3). Every product is stored semantically annotated with its position in the supermarket. Therefore, *product locator application* just needs to query those "coordinates" and draw the products in the supermarket map.

4.3 Supermarket Servers

The supermarkets count with two scopes for their servers:

- Internet, with global servers available from anywhere
- A particular supermarket, with servers placed in the supermarket itself

A survey performed with ALIMERKA (a Spanish located chain of supermarkets) for this research revealed that in their particular case they have a middle server located in the supermarket between the check-outs and the global servers located in their headquarters.

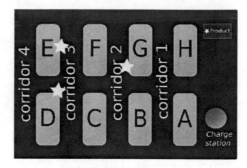

Fig. 3. Desired products marked on a supermarket plan

When users are at home defining what products they wish to buy, the *shopping cart application* will connect to the global servers of the chain of supermarkets. The retrieved information will contain global variables such as the name, price and code of the product. However, it will not contain information related to a particular supermarket.

Then, users in the supermarket will connect to both the global servers and the server located in the particular supermarket, which will contain information such as the current availability of the product in the supermarket (it may not be available in a supermarket as it would in bigger supermarkets; or it may not be in stock in that moment), or the location of products in the supermarket. The information available in each scope of the servers is summed in the table 1.

The communication of the different applications with the servers, and the synchronization among the servers is performed with Triple Spaces as detailed in section 4.4.

Table 1. Summary of the information provided by the different servers

Scope	Information	Description
	Name	The human readable name of the product
Global servers	Code	A unique identifier of the product
	Price	The price used in all the servers
Located servers	Location	Where is it in the supermarket (X,Y)?
	Availability	Is it sold here? Is it in stock?

4.4   Triple Spaces

TS is a paradigm which enables the coordination between processes deployed in heterogeneous devices writing and reading semantically described data in a shared space. The concrete TS solution we use is characterized by a full decentralization of the space through the nodes which joint it. In the described use case the different nodes are user's personal mobile phones, the supermarket's tablets, the chain of supermarket's global information management server and at least a server to manage the information of each specific supermarket (see Fig. 1).

This knowledge distribution is particularly interesting because the user information is written in his mobile device (section 4.1) fulfilling privacy issues. In any case, this information will become accessible by other nodes in the same space (i.e. *product locator application*), just when the user is connected to it.

4.5   Ontology

The ontology, which is dumped in the TS, is depicted in the Fig. 4. The most relevant concepts described by the ontology are:

Supermarket represents a concrete supermarket which belongs to a chain of supermarkets.

Product represents a concrete product sold by the chain of supermarkets.

ProductInSupermarket indicates if a specific product is sold in a given supermarket and its position. This information is required to locate a product in the mobile application map (see Fig. 3).

ShoppingCart represents the products the user wants to buy.

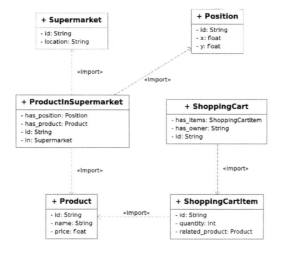

Fig. 4. Supermarket ontology

5   Conclusions and Further Work

This paper explores the use of a product locator application to enhance the shopping experience of people with mobility problems at supermarkets (such as handicapped or the elderly). The infrastructure used is fully decoupled and runs in mobile devices keeping the information of the user inside the boundaries of their personal devices.

In the future a robot will be responsible of guiding users, avoiding some issues such as security concerns related with the use of a supermarket's tablet. Moreover, the map will only be displayed as an alternative to the physical guiding of the robot, in those cases where supermarket is too crowded or the battery level is low.

Finally, an exhaustive evaluation of the final scenario is planned to be carried out. Similarly, the TS solution briefly described in this paper will be tested both in a heavily instrumented deployment scenario and using simulation tools.

Acknowledgments. This work has been supported by project grant TSI-020301-2009-27 (ACROSS), funded by the Spanish Ministerio de Industria, Turismo y Comercio.

References

1. Menus for the postmodern milieu (2010), http://www.boston.com/business/technology/articles/2010/10/24/menus_for_the_postmodern_milieu/
2. Ambient Assisted Living Joint Program (2011), http://www.aal-europe.eu/
3. Fensel, D.: Triple-Space Computing: Semantic Web Services Based on Persistent Publication of Information. In: Aagesen, F.A., Anutariya, C., Wuwongse, V. (eds.) INTELLCOMM 2004. LNCS, vol. 3283, pp. 43–53. Springer, Heidelberg (2004)
4. Gómez-Goiri, A., Emaldi, M., López-de-Ipiña, D.: A semantic resource oriented middleware for pervasive environments. UPGRADE journal (2011)
5. Krummenacher, R., Blunder, D., Simperl, E., Fried, M.: An open distributed middleware for the semantic web. In: International Conference on Semantic Systems, I-SEMANTICS (2009)
6. Nixon, L.J., Simperl, E., Krummenacher, R., Martin-Recuerda, F.: Tuplespace-based computing for the semantic web: a survey of the state-of-the-art. The Knowledge Engineering Review 23(02), 181–212 (2008)
7. Palazzi, C., Teodori, L., Roccetti, M.: Path 2.0: A participatory system for the generation of accessible routes. In: 2010 IEEE International Conference on Multimedia and Expo (ICME), pp. 1707–1711 (2010)
8. Walker, A.: Ageing in europe - challenges and consequences. Zeitschrift f r Gerontologie und Geriatrie 32(6) (1999)

Distributed Tracking System for Patients with Cognitive Impairments

Xabier Laiseca[1], Eduardo Castillejo[1], Pablo Orduña[1], Aitor Gómez-Goiri[1],
Diego López-de-Ipiña[1], and Ester González Aguado[2]

[1] Deusto Institute of Technology - DeustoTech
University of Deusto
Avda. Universidades 24, 48007 Bilbao, Spain
{xabier.laiseca,eduardo.castillejo,
pablo.orduna,aitor.gomez,dipina}@deusto.es
http://www.morelab.deusto.es
[2] Unidad de Investigación, Fundació Sant Antoni Abat (ABAT)
Hospital de Sant Antoni Abat - Consorci Sanitari del Garraf
c/ Sant Josep 21-3
08800 Vilanova i la Geltrú
egonzalez@fhcsaa.cat
http://www.fhcsaa.cat

Abstract. The increase of life expectancy has arisen new challenges
related with the amount of resources required to attend elderly people
with cognitive disabilities. These requirements, such as medical staff and
financial resources, have been multiplied in the last years, and this ten-
dency will continue in the forthcoming ones. In order to reduce these requirements, the introduction of new technologies will be a key aspect. In
this paper we propose a test-question-based memory game that collects
the answers given by patients and facilitates access to this information
to caregivers and relatives.

Keywords: cognitive impairments, memory game, elderly, triple space.

1 Introduction

The ageing of the population during the last decades has caused a substantial
growth of cognitive limitations cases in people, such as Alzheimer and dementia.
Moreover, the expected raise of the life expectancy suggests that the amount
of people affected by this kind of disabilities will be significantly increased [12].
Thus, hospitals' and residences' staff requirements will become economically
unsustainable. In other to tackle this problem, the use of new technologies which
ease caregivers' duties will be a key aspect.

In this paper, we propose a distributed system which is formed by two kinds
of nodes. The first node type is a memory game application used by patients
with cognitive disabilities. Therefore, to ease the interaction the game has been
designed taking into account the impairments of the users. This game is going to

J. Bravo, R. Hervás, and V. Villarreal (Eds.): IWAAL 2011, LNCS 6693, pp. 49–56, 2011.

be deployed in several nodes. The second one is a Web application that gathers the results obtained by the patients. This application can be used by patients' therapists and relatives.

Although the use of distributed architectures offers several benefits, it also raises new drawbacks. When facing this system the most relevant ones were: a) how to manage the information's flow (mainly the results of the patients), b) where to store the information, c) how to react to node crashes and d) how to add a new node without reconfiguring the whole system. In order to solve these issues, an architecture based on the Triple Space (TS) paradigm [4] has been used, which offers seamless solutions to these conflicts.

The rest of the paper is organized as follows. In Section 2 we discuss the related work. Section 3 explains the use case of the system. Section 4 describes the technical aspects of the proposed solution. Finally, Section 5 concludes this paper.

2   Related Work

With ageing of Europe [14], the infrastructures used for treating the elderly will gain relevance, and the costs of these infrastructures will increase notably. In order to optimize the costs of these infrastructures, the development of new technical solutions is required. In fact, the European Union is working in the promotion of programmes to develop applications and frameworks that enable the reduction of related costs and the increasing of factors that ease the quality of life of the elderly. Within this context, Ambient Assisted Living [1] solutions are arising across Europe to tackle these costs.

It has been proved that the use of videogames and new technologies ("serious games") can be useful as a support for the psychotherapy [3], as a tool in the physical rehabilitation after a stroke [10], and as a instrument of cognitive stimulation in Alzheimer patients [2,13]. In the case of dementia patients, the use of psychosocial programs of non-pharmacological intervention (cognitive behavioural therapy, elderly caregiver training, context adaptation, occupational therapy, activities and physical exercise programs, cognitive stimulation) have demonstrated to improve one or more aspects of the quality of life [8].

The use case presented in this paper is formed by several independent nodes which share their information. In order to share it in a very decoupled but expressive way TS paradigm is used. TS comes from tuplespace-based coordination languages where the interaction between processes is performed sharing information in a common space. Although, several approaches in the field of semantic tuplespaces exist [7,9], to the best of our knowledge this kind of solution has never been specifically designed and implemented to capture the dynamic and heterogeneous nature of future hospitals' network [6].

3   Use Case

As we detail in the system architecture section we have developed two different applications. The first one is a questionnaire game that patients will have to fill out. These questions are developed by therapists and the results are added to a historic. The other allows therapists to see and analyse patients' results. Next we describe the stakeholders' interactions with the presented system:

- Firstly, patients will have to login into the system in order to avoid results inconsistency. This task will be able to be made either by patients or caregivers, since we know that those patients may be elders or people with cognitive problems, which usually have interaction difficulties. A list of patients names will be presented, so just clicking on a name will allow the system to register them. We realized it became relevant to have multiple instances of the game running independently. With the given solution more than one patient can complete exercises in different nodes at the same time.

  Since there are some studies and previous works in face recognition and gestures capturing areas which can ease the login task [3,5], it is not the goal of our system.

- Thus, each patient will have to answer a few number of customized questions, as shown in Fig. 1, with different difficulty levels. These answers will allow therapists to analyse and manage their memory or cognitive progressions.

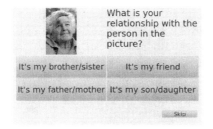

Fig. 1. Questionnaire window

- When the patient finishes the exercise, her answers are added to the historic stored in the space with additional data (e.g. username, current date, questions difficulty levels, correct answers taking into account these levels, etc.).
- On the other hand, therapists can analyse patients historical results. To that end, they will have to log into the system, and then they will be able to see the desired results. The developed web application displays patients' results and today's results. It also allows therapists to search for patients. Once a therapist selects one option the system generates a query which consults in the space for the desired information.
- As therapists can see patients results in their desktop application, patients' families will be able to do the same in their mobile devices (Fig. 2(a)).

It is expected that the usage of the presented technological solution, which enables therapists to remotely track results of users in the exercises will benefit the different actors at the following three levels:

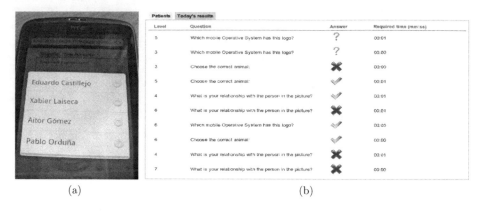

(a)   (b)

Fig. 2. Adapted interfaces to (a) mobile devices and (b) common desktop screens

- For the patients, the programs can be automatically adapted to their particular requirements at any moment. It generates ecological validity of the platform, improves the user satisfaction and increases the use of non-pharmacological treatments avoiding program abandonment.
- For the professionals, they can easily track patients online without requiring to wait for the results at the end of the program. This tracking will enable to perform customized adjustments of the exercises program taking into account the performance of the individual, adjusting the tasks with different levels of difficulty. It generates an efficiency improvement in the cognitive intervention programs, increases the use satisfaction of professionals and improves the cost-effectiveness relationship of these interventions.
- Finally, integrating caregivers and relatives to use these technologies improves the validity and trust of the data. Their implication makes them co-participants in the patient intervention plan, facilitates the communication among patients and professionals, and prevents burn-out effects on caregivers, which mostly results in the renunciation of the proper care.

This solution is built within the ACROSS project[1] (TSI-020301-2009-27), funded by the Spanish Ministerio de Industria, Turismo y Comercio. The project aims to incorporate robotic services into social scenarios allowing them to anticipate to user needs by improving communication and empathy between people and embodied agents. Although this is a first approach, more efforts are being placed for this solution to work out and to adapt to a robot in the Hospital de Sant Antoni Abat in Barcelona.

4   System Architecture

Due to the presented use case we have developed two different applications:

---
[1] http://www.acrosspse.com

– A desktop application was required in order to capture the patients' results. We called it Memory Game (Fig. 1) and its only purpose is to help patients to train their memory by a questionnaire. It has been developed in JavaSE using the SWT library[2], which is an open source widget toolkit for Java, providing a native look and feel to the applications. Designed user interfaces have been developed taking into account that patients may have some interaction difficulties or problems.

– A web application for therapists to consult all patients' results. This application has been developed using the Google Web Toolkit[3] (GWT) open source development toolkit, which basically allows developers to build and optimize complex web applications using the Java language. Thanks to GWT we can adapt its user interface in the browser to adapt itself for procuring the best suitability for mobile devices. This way, not only therapist would study patients results but their relatives could do it from their homes.

Both applications communicate each other by publishing and querying the TS. Memory Game will write on it every result for each patient. On the other hand, the GWT web application will launch some requests or queries to the space for receiving patients results.

Fig. 3 shows the information flow among the nodes connected to the TS.

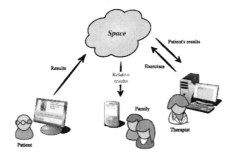

Fig. 3. System architecture and data sharing

4.1 Memory Game

The Memory Game is a desktop application for asking test questions to the patients. The asked questions can be private, such as "What is your relationship with the person in the picture?", or general knowledge questions, such as "Which is the animal of the photograph?". This questions are selected depending on a difficulty level preconfigured for each patient.

Because the patients of the game are elderly people, the user-friendliness is the application's main objective. In order to achieve it, the game has taken into account: a) designed to run in a touch screen to minimize the input/output devices to use, b) a reduced set of possible actions (choose user and answer) and c) a simple user interface that only uses text labels, big buttons and images.

---

[2] http://www.eclipse.org/swt/
[3] http://code.google.com/webtoolkit/

4.2   Results Web

The Results Web is the component responsible for listing patients and displaying the results of each one to therapists or to their relatives.

Therapists will probably use the application from the hospital's office desktop. However, familiars would very likely run the application in their mobile devices. In fact, nowadays it is claimed that around 40% of iPhone users browse the Web more frequently from their mobile device than from a desktop [11]. This can probably be applied to users of other smartphones (i.e. Android or Windows Phone devices) and this trend will probably increase in the near future.

By contrast, the Web is supported by most mobile devices. Some adaptation is required but only in the user interface, providing a proper layout, only the required contents, and avoiding plug-ins such as Adobe Flash or Java Applets.

Therefore, the technology selected to display results was the Web. The Results Web component is compounded by a servlet and a web client which communicates with the servlet through AJAX. The web client provides two different user interfaces (Fig. 2(b)), one adapted for the desktop, and the other adapted for mobile devices (Fig. 2(a)). Users will use any of these web interfaces and call methods provided by the servlet, which will act as a gateway to the TSs infrastructure.

Both the web client and the web server have been implemented in GWT, which is an open source technology developed by Google that provides an API to be used from the Java programming language. The toolkit is capable of translating that Java code to JavaScript. This way, a developer can use a Java IDE like Eclipse[4], and there write and test Java code, finally compiled into JavaScript.

4.3   Triple Spaces

The TS middleware used in the proposed solution allows the coordination between different processes writing and reading semantic information through a shared space easing the information's flow management. In the described use case, both the computers used by the patient and the web server which serves pages to mobile and normal clients are nodes from the same space.

Due to the decoupling nature of the middleware, the patients' computers or the web server do not depend on each other. Furthermore, no matter how many computers are used across the hospital by patients, the solution's behaviour will remain the same and additional configuration will not be required. As result of this capabilities and to the fact that TS allows to the developer to select where the information have to be stored, it facilitates the development of a error prone system which fulfils the challenges described in the introduction.

Moreover, the used middleware can be deployed on heterogeneous devices, so it could be possible to create a native mobile peer which does not act as a simple client of the web server. In this way, a central element or bottleneck such as the web server could be easily avoided or new applications could be easily developed to satisfy previously unidentified requirements.

---

[4] http://www.eclipse.org

4.4   Ontology

The ontology, which is dumped in the TS, is depicted in the Fig. 4. The most relevant concepts described by the ontology are:

User represents the user that can login in the system. The users can be therapists and patient's relatives.

Patient represents a patient of the hospital. The difficulty of the questions asked to a patient is defined by "min_level" and "max_level".

GameResult represents the questions done to a patient in a game play and the obtained results.

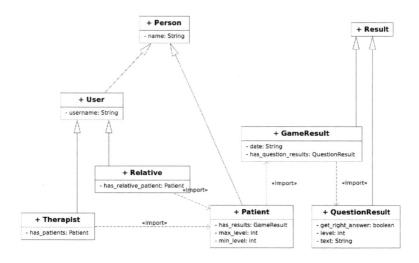

Fig. 4. System ontology

5   Conclusions and Further Work

In this paper, we presented a system that collects the patients' results of multiple nodes of the memory game application and offers these results to the patients' caregivers and relatives. To that end, we proposed a user-friendly solution which facilitates a) the interaction of elderly people and b) the caregivers' information gathering.

Our future plans include the deployment of the detailed system, as part of the ACROSS project, on a robotic platform. Once this deployment is finished, the proposed solution is going to be tested in a real environment by the research unit of the Sant Antoni Abat foundation. The target of this evaluation is to measure the impact on cognitive disability patients of these technologies.

Acknowledgments. This work has been supported by project grant TSI-020301-2009-27 (ACROSS), funded by the Spanish Ministerio de Industria, Turismo y Comercio.

References

1. Ambient Assisted Living Joint Program (2011), http://www.aal-europe.eu/
2. Barnes, D.E., Yaffe, K., Belfor, N., et al.: Computer-Based cognitive training for mild cognitive impairment: Results from a pilot randomized, controlled trial. Alzheimer Dis. Assoc. Disord. 23(3), 205–210 (2009)
3. Ceranoglu, T.: Video games in psychotherapy. Review of General Psychology 14(2), 141 (2010)
4. Fensel, D.: Triple-space computing: Semantic web services based on persistent publication of information. In: Aagesen, F.A., Anutariya, C., Wuwongse, V. (eds.) INTELLCOMM 2004. LNCS, vol. 3283, pp. 43–53. Springer, Heidelberg (2004)
5. Fernando, S., Money, A., Elliman, T., Lines, L.: Age Related Cognitive Impairments and Assistive Web-Base Technology
6. Gómez-Goiri, A., Emaldi, M., López-de-Ipiña, D.: A semantic resource oriented middleware for pervasive environments. UPGRADE Journal (2011)
7. Krummenacher, R., Blunder, D., Simperl, E., Fried, M.: An open distributed middleware for the semantic web. In: International Conference on Semantic Systems, I-SEMANTICS (2009)
8. Logsdon, R., McCurry, S., Teri, L.: Evidence-based interventions to improve quality of life for individuals with dementia. Alzheimer's Care Today 8(4), 309 (2007)
9. Nixon, L.J., Simperl, E., Krummenacher, R., Martin-Recuerda, F.: Tuplespace-based computing for the semantic web: a survey of the state-of-the-art. The Knowledge Engineering Review 23(02), 181–212 (2008)
10. Saposnik, G., Teasell, R., Mamdani, M., Hall, J., McIlroy, W.: Effectiveness of Virtual Reality Using Wii Gaming Technology in Stroke Rehabilitation. Stroke 41 (2010)
11. Sauer, F.: The enterprise apps in your pocket (2009), http://googlewebtoolkit.blogspot.com/2009/10/enterprise-apps-in-your-pocket.html
12. Steg, H., Strese, H., Loroff, C., Hull, J., Schmidt, S.: Europe Is Facing a Demographic Challenge Ambient Assisted Living Offers Solutions (March 2006)
13. Tárraga, L., Boada, M., Modinos, G., Espinosa, A., Diego, S., Morera, A., Guitart, M., Balcells, J., López, O., Becker, J.: A randomised pilot study to assess the efficacy of an interactive, multimedia tool of cognitive stimulation in Alzheimer's disease. British Medical Journal 77(10), 1116 (2006)
14. Walker, A.: Ageing in europe - challenges and consequences. Zeitschrift für Gerontologie und Geriatrie 32(6) (1999)

Designing Messenger Visual, an Instant Messaging Service for Individuals with Cognitive Disability

Pere Tuset[1], Juan Miguel López[2], Pere Barberán[1], Léonard Janer[1], and Cristina Cervelló-Pastor[3]

[1] Secció de Projectes de Transferència de Coneixement, TecnoCampus Mataró-Maresme, Av. Ernest Lluch 32, 08302 Mataró, Spain
{ptuset,barberan,leonard}@tecnocampus.cat
[2] Departamento de Lenguajes y Sistemas Informáticos, Universidad del País Vasco, C/Nieves Cano 12, 01006 Vitoria-Gasteiz, Spain
juanmiguel.lopez@ehu.es
[3] Departament d'Enginyeria Telemàtica, Universitat Politècnica de Catalunya, Av. Esteve Terradas 7, 08860 Castelldefels, Spain
cristina@entel.upc.edu

Abstract. Considering the importance of Internet-based communications in our society, the lack of Instant Messaging (IM) services adapted to individuals with cognitive disabilities who have difficulties using written language creates a situation of exclusion that has a negative impact on their daily lives. To alleviate this situation we present Messenger Visual, an IM service that uses pictograms as the main communication system. Along the paper we introduce the main design aspects of an IM service to support pictogram-based communications, as well as the design and evaluation aspects of an IM client that takes into account both the pictogram-based communication and the user interface accessibility requirements of individuals with cognitive disabilities.

Keywords: instant messaging services, augmentative and alternative communication, cognitive disability, user-centered design.

1 Introduction

Almost ten percent of the world's population lives with some type of disability [1]. One common aspect of disabled people is that they are prone to be excluded from society due to their condition. And despite the efforts being made to bridge the gap the exclusion situation is still far from being optimal, especially if we consider the digital society we are embracing. Today, albeit the shift from analog to digital technology has eliminated some accessibility barriers [2], individuals that live with a disability are also left apart from the digital society because most technology still fails to meet their accessibility requirements [3]. This situation needs to be addressed, as it reduces the independence of disabled individuals and causes social isolation.

Individuals with cognitive disabilities are one prime example of digital exclusion. Due to their condition they suffer from attention, memory and language impairments which difficult daily activities such as task planning and information processing [4].

J. Bravo, R. Hervás, and V. Villarreal (Eds.): IWAAL 2011, LNCS 6693, pp. 57–64, 2011.

But despite most of them are capable of using technological devices [5], the software that enables access to Internet services, such as browsers to access the World Wide Web (WWW), fails to take their requirements into account. For instance, the user interface of mainstream web browsers uses abstract concepts like tabs that are not easy to understand for such users. And other Internet services, such as electronic mail or instant messaging, are not in a better shape if we take into consideration that information in such media is usually presented in a textual format.

Nevertheless, this situation can be improved by developing user-centric software that takes into account the requirements of individuals with cognitive disabilities. This enables them to participate in the digital society [6], thus improving their independence and reducing social exclusion. For instance, the WWAAC (World Wide Augmentative and Alternative Communication) project [7] developed a WWW browser that uses pictogram-based Alternative and Augmentative Communication (AAC) to represent the information. But, to our knowledge, nowadays there is no single Instant Messaging (IM) service that meets the communication and user interface requirements of individuals with cognitive disabilities.

In this paper we present Messenger Visual, an IM service that enables individuals with cognitive disability to communicate over the Internet. The main differential aspect of Messenger Visual is that it replaces textual messages with pictograms-based messages, while providing the basic functionality of an IM service. We have also developed an IM client that takes into account the user interface accessibility requirements of individuals with cognitive disabilities. Finally, we have also evaluated the IM client using a user-centered approach, where users with cognitive disability have tested Messenger Visual as a regular activity.

The rest of the paper is organized as follows. Section 2 provides background related to the topics of the paper, namely Instant Messaging and Augmentative and Alternative Communications. Section 3 presents the design of a pictogram-based IM service to enable people with cognitive disability to communicate over the Internet. Section 4 presents the design of a pictogram-based IM client using a user-centered approach. Finally, Section 5 states the conclusions outlined from the development and evaluation of the project, and identifies the work that remains to be done in the future.

2   Related Work

IM services [8] are designed to enable users to exchange near real-time presence information and text-based messages over a public network, usually the Internet, to communicate with their contacts. In general, IM services rely on a client-server architecture to operate; IM servers provide features such as user access control and message routing, whereas IM clients provide a graphical interface for users to communicate. Nevertheless, IM services have evolved and now provide many other features besides the ones used for text-based communication, such as audio and video conferencing, file transfers and shared desktop.

Today most IM services are run by Internet-based companies, such as AOL, Yahoo and Microsoft. The protocols that support such IM services, as well as the software that enables users to communicate, are proprietary and their specifications are not publicly available. To provide with an open alternative the IETF

(Internet Engineering Task Force) had different groups dedicated to Internet-based IM services, obtaining a general model which was later adopted by two IM protocols, namely SIMPLE (SIP for Instant Messaging and Presence LEveraging) and XMPP (eXtensible Messaging and Presence Protocol). SIMPLE provides a set of extensions to SIP (Session Initiation Protocol) to support IM services, whereas XMPP derives from Jabber, an IM protocol based on XML (eXtensible Markup Language) which was initially designed by the open-source community [9].

Augmentative and Alternative Communications (AAC) [10] is a set of methodologies aimed at complementing or replacing written or spoken communications for those individuals that have such abilities impaired, either temporarily or permanently, due to injury or illness. One form of AAC are pictogram-based communication systems, which are built upon drawings or images that represent real objects or abstract concepts to enable individuals sharing internal states, feelings, ideas and experiences. Communication using pictograms usually consists of individuals selecting elements from a set of possibilities with the aid of an Assistive Technology (AT), which can either be low or high technology (i.e. a cardboard, a personal communicator or a computer).

Nowadays, there are many different pictogram-based communication systems, which are usually classified according to the transparency level of its pictograms; the level of resemblance between the pictograms and the objects or concepts they represent [10]. For instance, Rebus is a pictogram-based language developed by Woodcok to teach reading to children. PIC (Picture Ideogram Communication) was developed by Maharaj and its main characteristic is that they have a reverse contrast, i.e. white on black. Blissymbols was developed by Karl Blitz and is based on the ideographs of Chinese writing. Finally, PCS (Picture Communication Symbols) was developed by Roxana Mayer-Johnson and today it is one of the most widely used thanks to its transparency level.

3   Design of a Pictogram-Based Instant Messaging Service

This section presents the design of Messenger Visual, an IM service that uses pictograms as the main communication system. Like any other IM service, Messenger Visual shall support all the basic IM features [8], such as creating user accounts and logging in to the service, as well as adding/removing contacts, sending/receiving presence updates and sending/receiving messages to/from users in the contact list. To implement the basic IM features of Messenger Visual we use XMPP (eXtensible Messaging and Presence Protocol) [11] because it is based on standards and provides a decentralized client-server architecture that is flexible, scalable and secure. But the fact that Messenger Visual has to support pictograms as the main communication system adds additional requirements to the IM service. These requirements, together with the methodology to integrate them into the IM service, are described below.

The first requirement of a pictogram-based IM service is that users shall have a pictogram set available to communicate. To support such requirement there are two alternatives; having a personalized set of pictograms for each user or having a pictogram set that is shared among all users. The former approach allows pedagogues to define exactly which pictograms each user should have and to tailor it according to their learning process, whereas the latter approach gives more freedom to the user as they have the chance to access all the pictograms to communicate. Nevertheless, both approaches have drawbacks. On the one hand, having a personalized pictogram set may limit conversations between users as specific pictograms might not be available to some individuals. On the other hand, including a complete pictogram set may have a negative impact on interactivity, as users might need to spend more time browsing for pictograms to compose a message. But considering that actual trends in pictogram-based communication state that AAC (Augmentative and Alternative Communications) users should have a full set of pictograms available to communicate in order to promote their independence and support their learning process we decided, together with pedagogues, to have a shared pictogram set among all users.

Taking into account that pedagogues should be able to select the pictographic system that is most suitable to users according to their personal preferences and previous knowledge, the second requirement of a pictogram-based IM service is that it shall remain independent of the pictographic system that users employ to communicate. Furthermore, considering that elements within the pictographic system include both graphical and textual representation of the pictogram itself, the IM service shall also remain independent of the textual representation of such pictograms. To satisfy this design requirement we have developed an XML-based syntax that is able to represent pictogram-based messages unequivocally. Despite the fact that both XML and JSON (JavaScript Object Notation) are platform and language neutral, we have decided to use the former instead of the latter because it has better support for internationalization, i.e. textual representation of Chinese characters, and parsers are readily available. The XML syntax, shown in Figure 1, defines that each pictogram-based message is represented by a message element, which may contain one or more pictogram elements to represent pictograms within the message.

```
<message from="carolnogueras@messengervisual.net" to="isaacfernandez@messengervisual.net">
    <pictogram id="34" category="beings" text="you" />
    <pictogram id="67" category="actions" text="go" />
    <pictogram id="82" category="places" text="cinema" />
    <pictogram id="54" category="time" text="tonight" />
    <pictogram id="29" category="questions" text="question_mark" />
</message>
```

Fig. 1. Pictogram-based message representation using XML. A message element has a source and a destination and is composed of one or more pictogram elements. Each pictogram element contains a unique identifier, as well as the category it belongs to and the text associated to it.

Finally, considering that the vocabulary included in the pictogram set may change over time, the third requirement of a pictogram-based IM service is that it shall provide pedagogues with means for updating it. Two alternatives have been considered regarding the architecture to enable automatic pictogram updates; a centralized and a distributed approach. In the centralized architecture the pictogram set is stored in a server and retrieved by IM clients on demand. In contrast, in the distributed architecture each IM client has a local copy of the pictogram set that is synchronized with the server. In spite of requiring an additional synchronization mechanism, as pictogram set updates need to be notified to IM clients, we have decided to use a distributed architecture because it reduces the network bandwidth requirements as pictograms are cached at the IM client. To implement the pictogram set we use a relational database instead of separate files organized into folders because it is easier to maintain and offers performance advantages [12]. Finally, the protocol to enable pictogram database synchronization is based on XMPP to distribute update notifications among IM clients and HTTP (HyperText Transfer Protocol) to retrieve the pictogram database from the server, as represented in Figure 2.

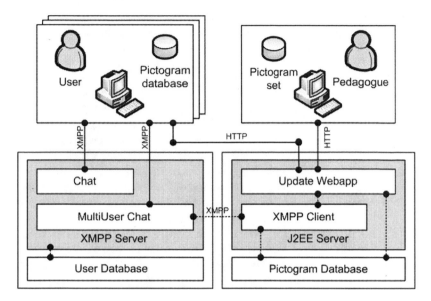

Fig. 2. Messenger Visual service architecture. XMPP supports the basic IM features, as well as pictogram-based communications and pictogram database update notifications. Whenever an update is triggered, IM clients download the pictogram database from the server using HTTP.

4   Design of a Pictogram-Based Instant Messaging Client

The next step to enable individuals with cognitive disabilities to communicate using the pictogram-based IM service is to develop an IM client that meets pictogram-based communication requirements. The IM client must provide a user interface that suits user requirements. As a first step, the requirements for a standard IM client were analyzed. In this sense, we found that the user interface of an IM client is organized to provide with a series of basic functionalities, such as access control, contacts management and chat conversations [8]. Although a first prototype of the IM client had already been implemented [13], it didn't completely meet the requirements of cognitively disabled users and, thus, required further analysis and development.

From this analysis we decided that the user interface should be organized with the same structure as a common IM client. Taking end user capabilities into account, the user interface should also be limited only to the strictly necessary elements to carry out the actions that users can perform in an IM service. Moreover, the user interface should be designed to be as simple as possible, avoiding the use of complex metaphors and without including hidden or implicit elements. In this sense, the user interface should be an almost completely visual interface. Written language might be included, but only as a support for social educators and users with some written language communication skills. Furthermore, elements in the user interface should be organized according to the requirements of the pictographic system, i.e. categories.

Albeit the IM service has been designed to remain independent from the pictographic system employed by users to communicate, we have initially decided to use a specific pictogram set as the IM client is to be evaluated with users at Fundació El Maresme, a non-profit organization that intends to promote the social integration of users with intellectual or cognitive disability and their families. To decide which set of pictograms should be used, we considered that users are already familiar with PCS (Picture Communication Symbols) because they use a piece of software called Boardmaker [14] in their daily activities. But considering the fact that PCS pictograms are licensed, and taking into account that ARASAAC (ARAgoneSe portal of Augmentative and Alternative Communication) pictograms [15] are similar but licensed under a Creative Commons BY-NC-SA license, we have finally decided to implement ARASAAC as the pictographic system of Messenger Visual.

The design of the IM client using a user-centered approach with users from Fundació El Maresme was conducted in fortnightly one-hour-long sessions that lasted for six months. During the sessions users were located in different rooms to resemble physical distance and pedagogues and social educators were present. These sessions served to evaluate the IM client in order to provide feedback about its possible shortcomings. After some iteration in the user interface design process, a first fully functional prototype that met all of the abovementioned requirements was developed.

To enforce access control the IM client is based on two different windows, as shown in Figure 3. First of all, the login window allows users to select their profile from a matrix of local user profiles stored in the computer. The window also offers a mechanism to create a new user account or to add an existing account to the local user profiles. Once users have selected their profile they must provide their passphrase in the password window to log in. Considering usability requirements the passphrase is based on a combination of four numeric digits represented by pictograms.

Once users have logged in, a window to manage contacts appears. The window contains a list with all the contacts that are currently online and is updated whenever a contact logs in or logs out. Taking into account usability requirements, the contacts in the list are represented by the user picture and full name. The contact window also provides a mechanism to add and remove contacts from the list. To start a new conversation with a contact from the list a user has to click on the contact picture.

Last but not least, the chat window allows users to communicate by means of exchanging pictogram-based messages. According to the ARASAAC pictogram organization, the top of the interface contains the categories in which pictograms are classified. On the left side the most frequent pictograms appear in order to ease the composition of common messages (i.e. *Hello, Goodbye, Yes, No* and *Thank you*). On the right side the pictograms that belong to the active category are displayed. On the bottom lies the pictogram input space to compose a message. Finally, the central part of the window contains the actual conversation that the user is having.

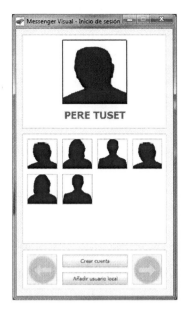
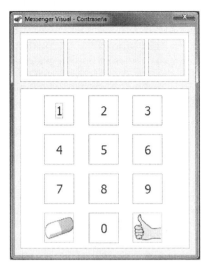

Fig. 3. Messenger Visual client user interface. The login window enables individuals to select their profile using a picture from the local user profile matrix, whereas the password window enables users to type in their four-digit numeric passphrase using pictograms.

5   Conclusions and Future Work

This paper has presented Messenger Visual, an IM service that enables individuals with cognitive disability to communicate over the Internet using pictogram-based messages. Along the text we have described and discussed the decisions to make Messenger Visual support the basic requirements of an IM service, as well as how we have enabled support for pictogram-based communications. We have also presented an IM client adapted to the requirements of individuals with cognitive disability and we have evaluated it using a user-centric approach. The evaluation has provided feedback that indicates that cognitively disabled individuals are able to communicate using pictograms, thus enabling social interaction and promoting digital inclusion.

Nevertheless, during the evaluation we have detected that some parts of the IM client user interface might need to be changed in order to increase usability. Some elements present a functionality that can be interpreted in different ways, thus becoming a source of possible confusion to users. For instance, buttons to navigate the contact list at the contact window operate in an up and down fashion, whereas buttons to navigate categories and pictograms in the chat window operate in a left and right fashion. Despite we have not observed important difficulties using such interface elements during the evaluation, we believe that redesigning those elements to provide more consistency will lead to an interface that is more usable by individuals.

Finally, all the knowledge we have today about how individuals with cognitive disability use Messenger Visual is based on qualitative research methods, such as interviews and ethnography. Thus, we are developing a tool to automatically collect and process statistical information about how users interact with the IM client user interface to communicate. For instance, we plan to explore parameters such as the average number of pictograms per message or the percentage of pictograms that users require in a conversation. This information, collected over time, will provide a deeper understanding of how users with cognitive disability communicate using pictograms.

References

1. World Health Organization. World report on disability,
   `http://www.who.int/disabilities/world_report/concept_note_`
   `2010.pdf`
2. Atkinson, R., Castro, D.: Digital Quality of Life: Understanding the Personal and Social Benefits from the Information Technology Revolution. In: Information Technology and Innovation Foundation (October 2008)
3. Glinert, E., York, B.: Computers and People with Disabilities. ACM Transactions on Accessible Computing 1(2) (October 2008)
4. LoPrestri, E., Bodine, C., Lewis, C.: Assistive Technology for Cognition: Understanding the Needs of Persons with Disabilities. IEEE Engineering in Medicine and Biology Magazine 27(2), 29–39 (2008)
5. Gregor, P., Dickinson, A.: Cognitive difficulties and access to information systems: an interaction design perspective. Journal of Universal Access to Information Society 5, 393–400 (2007)
6. Todis, B., Sohlberg, M., Hood, D., Fickas, S.: Making electronic mail accessible: Perspectives of people with acquired cognitive impairments, caregivers and professionals. Brain Injury Journal 19(6), 389–401 (2005)
7. Poulson, D., Nicolle, C.: Making the Internet accessible for people with cognitive and communication impairments. Universal Access Information Society 3(1), 48–56 (2004)
8. Jennings, R., Nahum, E., Olshefski, D., Saha, D., Shae, Z., Waters, C.: A Study of Internet Instant Messaging and Chat Protocols. IEEE Network, 16–21 (July/August 2006)
9. Saint-Andre, P.: Streaming XML with Jabber/XMPP. IEEE Internet Computing, 82–89 (September/October 2005)
10. Glennen, S., DeCoste, D.: Handbook of Augmentative and Alternative Communication. Singular Publishing Group, San Diego (1998)
11. IETF. Extensible Messaging and Presence Protocol: Core (RFC3920),
    `http://tools.ietf.org/pdf/rfc3920.pdf` (last accessed on January 7, 2011)
12. Sears, R., van Ingen, C., Gray, J.: To BLOB or Not To BLOB: Large Object Storage in a Database or a Filesystem? Technical Report (June 2006)
13. Tuset, P., Barberán, P., Janer, L., Delgado, S., Buscà, E., Vilà, N.: Messenger Visual: A pictogram-based IM service to improve communications among disabled people. In: NordiCHI 2010: 6th Nordic Conference on Human-Computer Interaction, pp. 797–800 (October 2010)
14. Mayer-Johnson: Boardmaker Software Family,
    `http://www.mayer-johnson.com/products/boardmaker-software/`
15. Aragonese Portal of Augmentative and Alternative Communication (ARASAAC),
    `http://www.catedu.es/arasaac/`

ATHENA: Smart Process Management for Daily Activity Planning for Cognitive Impairment

Eva Hidalgo[1], Luis Castillo[1], R. Ignacio Madrid[2], Óscar García-Pérez[1],
M.R. Cabello[1], and J. Fdez-Olivares[3]

[1] IActive Intelligent Solutions, Granada, Spain
{E.Hidalgo,L.Castillo,O.Garcia,M.Cabello}@iactive.es
[2] Instituto de Innovación para el Bienestar Ciudadano, Málaga, Spain
nmadrid@i2bc.es
[3] University of Granada
Faro@decsai.ugr.es

Abstract. Smart Process Management is a technology, based on Artificial Intelligence planning and scheduling, able to design timed sequences of activities that solve a problem in a given environment. In the framework of Ambient Assisted Living, it is being used for decision support for the daily care of patients with cognitive impairment, either for the patient themselves or for their care givers or senior care center staff by designing personalized daily activity plans for the specific case of every patient or the resources available at senior care centers.

1 Introduction

ATHENA is a pilot application that shows how IActive Smart Process Management technologies (SPM here on) provides added value decision support for the daily care of patients with cognitive impairment, either for the patient themselves or for their care givers or senior care center staff, introducing a new dimension in the enabling technologies for the ageing well.

AAL systems need to evolve to meet the requirements of individuals as their needs and circumstances change [9]. Current AAL environments are very rich in sensing capabilities and they are even able to infer the state of subjects, the task they are doing, carry out diagnostic processes, etc [7]. However, once the critical information is collected they frequently lack of the capability to suggest complex (non structured) goal-oriented behaviors. ATHENA tries to go a step beyond by using SPM technology to adapt general and clinical guidelines to design daily or weekly activity and care plans for patients with cognitive impairments, adapted to their cognitive state, their care requirements, their preferences or needs. These plans, that may be edited and modified in an interactive process, may be used with two different purposes,

- For patients and their care givers, these plans may be used to structure the evolution of the day, to monitor the activities as they are carried out, to detect meaningful deviations and to help patients by providing alternative ways to resume their activity.

J. Bravo, R. Hervás, and V. Villarreal (Eds.): IWAAL 2011, LNCS 6693, pp. 65–72, 2011.

– For senior care centers or organizations, ATHENA also enables their technical staff to arrange the available resources (e.g. nurses, physicians, physiotherapists, monitors, rooms, laboratories, etc) and coordinate them with the offer of scheduled activities and the set of patients in the center or at home, respecting their shifts and their duty periods.

From an ICT point of view, ATHENA is a simple web application, although it embodies very sophisticated Artificial Intelligence and SPM technologies to provide the functionality described above. One of the most outstanding features of ATHENA is its ease of use either for patients or technical staff. Both of them are completely unaware of being using sophisticated artificial intelligence technology just by easily pointing and clicking on a simple screen button (we are working on a new version in which patients interact with a interactive virtual agent [6]).

2   Users' Perspective

Elderly people frequently suffer from different physical and mental conditions related to the aging process. One of the most disruptive ones is cognitive impairment, that affect memory as well as other essential cognitive functions (attention, language, reasoning, etc). Cognitive impairments varies in its severity (from mild cognitive impairment to more serious impairments related to Dementia or Alzheimer disease) and tend to deteriorate as time passes impacting not only in the health status but also in the persons' ability to plan and perform daily life activities normally [8].

Currently, elderly people suffering from cognitive impairments have different options to receive care: they can stay at home with the support of informal and formal carers, attend to senior day care centers or move to respite or residential care homes. In all these cases, different people (family, nurses and/or therapists) take the responsibility to plan and monitor the care and daily activities of the elderly, . This is a dynamic and complex task, since users' needs may change by the interaction between the normal course of deterioration on cognitive functioning and the results of medical or care treatments. As a consequence, the care/activities plans for each patient have to be personalized and updated continuously in order to maximize their effectiveness.

This scenario requires the organization and allocation of the existing resources and frequently impose a burden both at personal and organizational level. At personal level, family and professional carers may suffer of what is called the care givers' burnout syndrome. At organizational level, there are limited economic and professional resources which allocation has to be optimized.

From this users' perspective, the question that ATHENA addresses is how multiple personal and physical resources can be managed effectively in order to organize the care and daily activities of people suffering from cognitive impairments based on their specific needs.

3   Description of the ATHENA System

3.1   Introduction to Smart Process Management Technology

Reasoning systems have been recognized as one of the key enabling technologies in the field of AAL [10]. These systems represent, analyze and conclude knowledge about users' state and the context situation in order to take a decision.

In this context, the project presented here is based in IActive Smart Process Management technology, a proactive intelligent technology for decision support that allows to use expert knowledge to design a sequence of activities for solving a given problem. In general, SPM allows to represent expert knowledge, the skills and the expertise of real experts to handle different instances of problems. This knowledge is modeled in a form understandable by the core of the technology: the smart process manager. The smart process manager interprets the description of every problem, applies the expert knowledge and finds a way to solve the problem.

SPM technology, created in and transferred from the University of Granada [1], has also been used within apparently different areas like tourism [2], civil [4] and military emergency management, pediatric oncology [5] or e-learning [3], among others. SPM technology is a proactive intelligent technology for decision support that allows to use expert knowledge to design a sequence of activities for solving a given problem. In general, SPM allows to represent expert knowledge, the skills and the expertise of real experts to handle different instances of problems. This knowledge is modeled in a form understandable by the core of the technology: the smart process manager. The smart process manager interprets the description of every problem, applies the expert knowledge and finds a way to solve the problem. In the case of ATHENA, a problem is the design of a daily/weekly activity plan for cognitively disabled patients personalizing the plan to the features of every patient and to the available resources in his/her environment.

The workbench of the technology (see Figure 1) is IActive Knowledge Studio, a tool for modeling the knowledge associated to a problem and for delivering intelligent components, based on SPM technology. Knowledge Studio has been used to develop the intelligent core of ATHENA within the following life cycle:

1. A representation of the knowledge about the environment: profiles and features of the patients, available activities and their schedule, features and available resources of the center, etc.
2. Knowledge Studio also allows for representing the expert knowledge required to solve problems in the form of general and clinical guidelines.
3. From these inputs, the smart process manager, named IActive Decisor, analyzes the applicable guidelines, adapt them to both the cognitive state of every patient, their requirements, their needs and even their preferences but also to the available activities and resources of a given senior center to design a customized daily/weekly activities plan.
4. Physicians may revise the plan, add, remove activities or request a new design of the plan.

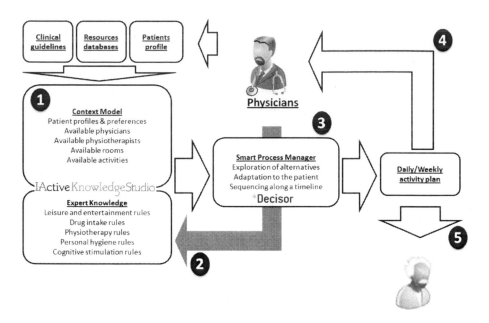

Fig. 1. Life cycle of the application of Smart Process Management Technology (Decisor)

5. Once the plan is approved by the physician, it may be communicated to every patient or care giver to structure the development of the daily activities.

3.2   Description of ATHENA Knowledge Base

ATHENA assumes that all the patients under treatment are hosted in a senior care center, but it could be extended to home care situations easily. This senior care center has a set of resources (nurses, physicians, physiotherapists, monitors, rooms, laboratories, etc) and a scheduled offer of activities. Every patient must follow its treatment and he/she has assigned a set of activities (personal care, drug intake, leisure and entertainment, physiotherapy, physician revision, training, etc) depending on his/her specific case and adapted to the schedule of the center. Al this information is stored in ATHENA's knowledge database. This knowledge base of ATHENA, as it is encoded in Knowledge Studio, is divided into two sections, the Context Model, which describe the environment of the problem, and the Expert Knowledge, that describes the expertise and the existing guidelines about how to organize an activity plan.

Knowledge About the Environment. The Context Model contains, among other, the information about the following items and the relations among them.

1. Patients. Name, gender, age and other bureaucratic information, their cognitive level, and statistical data about their planned activities.

2. Staff. Identification data, their timetable and their skills and availability.
3. Center timetable. The regular time intervals which structure the activities along the day (breakfast, mid morning, lunch, etc).
4. Available activities. Type of activity, requirements (cognitive level, age, gender), schedule, resources and staff involved.

All this information is represented in UML 2.0, the Unified Modeling Language as it is shown in Figure 2(left).

Expert Knowledge. Expert knowledge represents the skills and experience gathered from human experts in solving known problems. Knowledge Studio allows to represent this information just by using four graphical constructs, as shown in Figure 2(right).

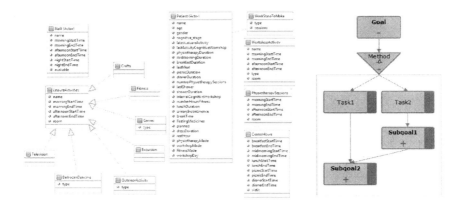

Fig. 2. (left) Main classes and their relationships in UML 2.0 as they are represented in the Context Model (right) Four basic graphical constructs of Expert Knowledge: compound *goals* that may be decomposed into one or more subgoals by following decomposition *methods*. A goal may be decomposed by following multiple, alternative methods and one or more subgoals may be *tasks* which are non-decomposable, primitive activities. All these elements are related by means of *arrows* to represent precedence constraints.

In ATHENA, the main goal of the Expert Knowledge is the design of the activities to be carried out by one or more patients within a given time horizon. Every patient is explored to select the most appropriate activities among all the available ones. The list of covered activities in the guidelines range in the following offer.

– Leisure and entertainment. Depend on the cognitive state of every patient. They range from watching TV (appropriate for persons with severe impairments) to petanque playing or excursions (for persons with a mild impairment).

- Drug intake is usually considered, unless there are other recommendations, after main meals, taking into account the timetable of the center. The possibility of assigning a monitor to support one or more patients during their meals is also considered in the ATHENA, depending on the cognitive state of every patient as well as the expected time required to finish the meal.
- When the center has set up a physiotherapy service, the physiotherapist(s) will be assigned a room and a timetable. The duration and the number of sessions depend on the cognitive state of patients. It has also been assumed that a physiotherapy session and a gym session cannot be assigned for the same patient the same day.
- Regarding personal hygiene, the cognitive state of the patient would lead to assign a smaller or greater time frame and to arrange the assistance of a monitor, depending on the timetable of monitors available in the center.
- Cognitive stimulation activities are also considered, up to physicians recommendations, and they are assigned to patients depending on their state and the availability of this activity in the center.

These activities are encoded as *goals* since they might be accomplished in different ways by following different decomposition methods, let say, depending on their cognitive state, age or gender.

3.3   Care and Activity Plans

When requested, IActive Decisor will explore the set of available guidelines in the Expert Knowledge, will connect to ATHENA's knowledge base to extract the data from the Context Model required to apply clinical guidelines both about patients profiles and about the resources available in the center. It then will explore patient's profiles and, as a result, will design a daily/weekly activity plan for every patient These plans contains details about the following items (among others):

1. How to carry out activity? Take into account interdependencies between activities, their start and end dates and their relative ordering.
2. Who carries out every activity? Identify staff and patients involved in every activity.
3. When an activity has to be carried out? Personalize the duration of every activity, taking into account shift of staff, scheduled activities.
4. Which resources are involved? Take into account available resources and staff and the organization rules of the center.

3.4   Implementation

Once the Context Model and the Expert Knowledge have been represented and validated within IActive Knowledge Studio, an intelligent module is delivered, either as a Java package or as a Web Service ready to be integrated into larger IT systems or to build a brand new application on top of it. ATHENA fits in the last case. It is a simple web application (see Figure 3, built on top of a web service that embraces the knowledge represented in Knowledge Studio and the IActive Decisor as its main search engine, and it also allows for displaying its resulting plans through any web browser.

This plan is sent back to ATHENA and it will be displayed through ATHENA graphical interface in any web browser. All this is just one "point and click" away in ATHENA's interface. It is worth saying that ATHENA not always suggest the same plan for the same patient, since it all depends on the context of the problem, state of patients and availability of resources.

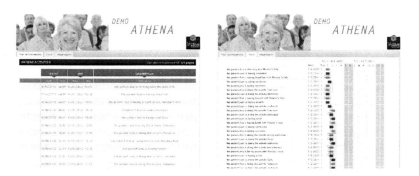

Fig. 3. Main screen of ATHENA showing the detailed plan (left) and a Gant Chart (right) for two patients obtained by Decisor

4   Conclusions

ATHENA enables care givers and senior care center's technical staff to take into account the profile of patients with cognitive impairments and the offer of activities and resources in order to design a customized activities plan for every patient (and therefore, for every center) providing an added value in ICT enabling technologies within Ambient Assisted Living frameworks. ATHENA is just a small web application to showcase the capabilities of IActive Smart Process Management technology and may be integrated into larger IT health care systems or be used as the basement for a brand new application on top of it. Among its most outstanding features, are the following ones:

- Patients will have a daily/weekly activities plan adapted to their features, preferences, needs and cognitive state.
- Care givers may track what every patient must be doing at any moment.

In more ambitious applications under consideration for future work, ATHENA framework might be enhanced with more funcionalities:

- ATHENA might be used to size up the number of services, activities and technical staff required for a senior center to develop its daily activity and even to optimize its staff according to the expected hosting of patients and their profiles.

- Wearable devices and sensors, or smartphones might also be considered to integrate and monitor these personal activity plans and launch customized reminders (either voiced, textual or visual) to follow the critical parts of the plan.
- Interactive Virtual Agents [6] may also be considered as a reinforcement for enabling a more efficient and easier to follow interface with patients. Depending on the severity of their impairments, interacting with these virtual agents might be likely the only possible way of interaction.

References

1. Castillo, L., Fdez-Olivares, J., García-Pérez, O., Palao, F.: Efficiently handling temporal knowledge in an HTN planner. In: Sixteenth International Conference on Automated Planning and Scheduling, ICAPS (2006)
2. Castillo, L., Armengol, E., Onaindía, E., Sebastiá, L., González-Boticario, J., Rodríguez, A., Fernández, S., Arias, J.D., Borrajo, D.: SAMAP. An user-oriented adaptive system for planning tourist visits. Expert Systems With Applications 35(2) (2008)
3. Castillo, L., Morales, L., González-Ferrer, A., Fdez-Olivares, J., Borrajo, D., Onaindía, E.: Automatic generation of temporal planning domains for e-learning problems. Journal of Scheduling 13(1), 347–362 (2010)
4. Fdez-Olivares, J., Castillo, L., García-Pérez, O., Palao, F.: Bringing users and planning technology together. experiences in SIADEX. In: Sixteenth International Conference on Automated Planning and Scheduling, ICAPS (2006); Awarded as the Best Application Paper of this edition
5. Fdez-Olivares, J., Castillo, L., Cózar, J.A., García-Pérez, O.: Supporting clinical processes and decisions by hierarchical planning and scheduling. Computational Intelligence (to appear)
6. Florencio, E., Amores, G., Pérez, G., Manchón, P.: Aggregation in the In–Home Domain. Procesamiento del lenguaje natural 40, 17–26 (2008)
7. Nugent, C.D., Augusto, J.C., Martin, S.: Towards personalization of services and an integrated service model for smart homes applied to elderly care. In: Proceedings of the International Conference on Smart Homes and Health Telematic
8. Landow, M.L.: Cognitive Impairment: Causes, Diagnosis and Treatment. Nova Sciece Publishers, Bombay (2010)
9. Dragone, M., Tynan, R., O'Grady, M.J., Muldoon, C., O'Hare, G.M.P.: Towards evolutionary ambient assisted living systems. Journal of Ambient Intelligence and Humanized Computing 1(1), 15–29 (2010)
10. van den Broek, G., Cavallo, F., Wehrmann, C.: AALIANCE. Ambient Assisted Living Roadmap. IOS Press, Amsterdam (2010)

RFID Performance in Localization Systems

Iván Álvarez, Pedro Malagón,
Marina Zapater, Juan-Mariano de Goyeneche, and José M. Moya

Dept. Ingeniería Electrónica
ETSI Telecomunicación
Universidad Politécnica de Madrid
{ivanam,malagon,marina,goyeneche,josem}@die.upm.es
http://www.elb105.es

Abstract. RFID (Radio Frequency Identification) is a technology widely
deployed in access control of particular and professional places. Within
this technology, individuals must carry a passive tag with them. When
the tag is inside the area of influence of a RFID reader, the exchange
information grant access to the carrier. As the individual must carry a
tag, it is possible to track the tag around the place, with more readers,
in order to provide more context information to an AAL (Ambient Assisted Living) system. While access applications can require interaction
from the user, localization systems are more successful if they are completely passive, with no interaction from the user. We first find out what
kind of tag is preferred in a concrete professional company. In addition
we experimentally evaluate the performance of preferred tags in different parts of the user (pocket, wallet, shirt-pocket, etc.). The experiment
try to find the distance that the reader can obtain the information from
the tag in different scenarios, and view the influence of human body
and metal over this read range, that we know are hostile enviroment.
Analyzing the results, we suggest considerations to implement a passive
RFID localization system: place the readers in vertical position (horizontal reading) and attach a non-metallic cover to the tag to guarantee a minimum separation between the tag and human body (minimum
of 2 mm).

1 Introduction

Ambient Intelligence (AmI) and Ambient Assisted Living (AAL) applications
require context information to help users in their daily life. Human activity is
an important part of contextual intelligence for ubiquitous human-centric services, such as health-care services. These applications need distributed sensors
to obtain as much information of the environment as possible. User-centric sensors are important to provide personalized reactions depending on the people
involved in an event. In order to achieve better performance in a sensing system,
superposition of sensors and technologies is advisable.

Radio Frequency Identification (RFID) is an important enabling technology for context-awareness in ubiquitous computing. Is one of the most used

J. Bravo, R. Hervás, and V. Villarreal (Eds.): IWAAL 2011, LNCS 6693, pp. 73–78, 2011.

technologies for physical grant access, and it is widely used in AmI or to develop AAL, where identification is one of the most important thing to do.

RFID technology has gained increasing attention as a low cost, flexible, and relatively fast solution for wireless identification [1]. RFID would support the development of new strategies for autonomic and home networking, mobility control, resource allocation, security, and service discovery algorithms [2].

There are several killer applications for RFID in the market nowadays: grant access in buildings, patient localization and identification in hospitals and equipment tracking [3], and several companies provide equipments and algorithms to deploy them, such as [4] or [5]. In each of these applications, the system manager decides where the tag must be set in order to the system.

In this paper, we analyze how RFID technology works under normal behavior of the users, who are already used to carry a RFID tag for grant access system.

In section 2 we present our motivation to study RFID performance as a localization system. In section 3 we describe the setup of the experiment and comment the results obtained. Finally, in section 4 we present the conclusions obtained from the experiment done.

2   Motivation

RFID allows contactless identification of objects using RF [6]. We believe that passive RFID is an interesting technology for supporting localization services. Its main advantages are lack of battery management, wireless localization, identification, accuracy in measurement. It is widely used for access control; for example, credit control in public transportation, building access depending on personal permission,...

Passive RFID has different working frequencies: LF (125KHz-148MHz), HF (13.56MHz), UHF (868MHz, 915MHz). The reader range is longer as the frequency increases, although it is more sensitive to liquid/metal interference. LF is typically used for animal identification. HF is typically used for access control. UHF is generally used for object/user tracking.

The RFID localization system we want to evaluate would be part of an Object Tracking System (OTS), such as the presented in [7]. Each RFID reader would be a clue injector of the system, providing reader power used, distance and identity of both reader and card. The system is compatible with other clue injectors, based in RFID (for example, [8]) or not.

There are a lot of proposals for localization services based on RFID ([9],[10], [11]). We focus on the reader range in different scenarios. Thus, liability of the service (rate of user detection) does not need to be 100%. We believe that the rate of use (users carrying the tag) is more important. Consequently, we have prepared a survey for workers in a electronic engineering laboratory, where 16 researchers, technicians and administration staff work everyday. They already use a HF RFID tag (short-distance MIFARE ISO14443 card [12]) for identification and access control. The goal of the survey is detect which option is better to use for indoor localization, taking into account that a different tag is needed (HF tag is not valid for UHF reader).

Table 1. Preference voting for possible tags

	Votes	Could	Against
UHF wristband + HF wristband	4	0	12
UHF wristband + HF card	5	0	11
UHF card + HF card	7	4	5
UHF sticker + HF card	11	2	3
Hanged UHF card + HF card	7	5	4
UHF card + HF wristband	2	1	13
Dual card	13	2	1

We can conclude that workers are used to carry a card with them and can tolerate carrying another extra-card. Most of them prefer to carry only one tag, either a dual card or a sticker in a previous deployed card. Users don't feel inclined to carry extra objects for location services, although they already did for access mechanisms. Access mechanisms have forced users to adapt to it, in order to enter in a room or building. As the localization system failure doesn't entail an immediate withdraw, users are less receptive to adapt themselves.

The option used in hospital systems, a wristband, is a priori not attractive for users.

Therefore, we decide to perform the experiments with traditional RFID cards, as is the main option for users.

3   Experiment

This experiment represents a possible implementation of a passive UHF RFID localization system. The reader is set inside the suspended ceiling, top-down oriented to read equally from any direction. The distance from ceiling to floor is 3 m. The experiment consists in reading some cards in different positions to view the influence of human body, metal and the presence of other antennas.

The reader used is DL920, distributed by Daily RFID [13], shown in Figure 1. It is a UHF reader (860 MHz to 960 MHz), supporting EPC Gen2 ISO18000-6B/6C protocol. The transmit power can be configured to a maximum of 30 dBm, in order to achieve a read distance between 8 m and 15 m (in perfect conditions of orientation and no interference).

We recreate different real situations to find out how the system adapts to them. The tag used is a standard RFID UHF card. We introduce the different conditions and table 2 shows the results obtained. First of all, we test a hanged card around the neck with different materials to hang it. The card can be hanged with a metal clip and with a non-metal clip. Moreover, the card can be covered with clothes or not. The behavior is different There are three different possibilities: hanged with a non-metal clip, with a metal clip and covered with some clothes.

Secondly, we introduced the card in a wallet, and carry it inside our clothes (in the shirt pocket) and closed to the human body (inside pant's pocket). In

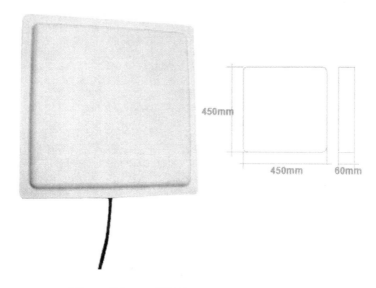

Fig. 1. DL920: UHF long distance reader

the first case, the reader is closer to the tag and the separation with the human body is greater, because this pocket is looser.

The distance shown in table 2 were calculated as the horizontal projection of the distance between reader and user.

Table 2. Reading distances

Case	Reading distance
Hanged without metal pin	3.7 meters
Hanged without metal pin and covered the card by some clothes	2.8 meters
Hanged with metal pin	1.75 meters
Wallet into pocket without contact	1.5 meters
Into wallet	2 meters
Hanged at waist outside pocket with a metal pin	1.7 meters

Finally, we check the compatibility with an existing system. As stated in the survey shown in table 1, two cards in the same place or a sticker in an existing HF card are the preferred options. Therefore, we test the separation needed between RFID cards.

From the measures done, we conclude that the best situation is using a card hanged with non-metal clip. It is the result expected, as the distance to the body is greater than other scenarios and there is no metal interference. If the user already has a HF tag hanged to grant access, it is mandatory separate both tags at least 4.4 mm. A plastic structure which keeps cards separated can be offered for a correct system. Avoiding overlap of cards to the maximum (having different hang-points, different corners) has the same response as the separation.

Table 3. Passive RFID card separation

Case	Minimum separation between elements
Cards working in different frequencies	4.4 mm
Cards that work in the same frequency	1.5 mm
Card and body	1.6 mm

Clothes over the card reduce reader range due to the smaller separation between body and card. If metal-zip clothes are used, the reader doesn't work properly.

The separation between body is also relevant when using a card inside the pocket, where the distance is smaller. When a wallet is used, it grants a separation to make it work. It works better in the shirt pocket, because separation and height is bigger.

4 Conclusions

Users who mandatory need a HF RFID tag for grant access applications prefer a compatible tag (such as another card or a sticker) rather than an extra tag (such as a wristband). With these tags, the correct reading depends on the distance, the antenna polarization, the power emission and antennas.

To check the suitability of the system we experimentally estimate the read range of a UHF passive tag (a card) from the reader in different real situations. The best situation to get the read range from a reader is, as expected, to use a card with no interfering elements. Direct contact with metal or human body reduce the read range and makes the system practically unfeasible. Metal-zip wallets and metal pens reduce efficiency. Related to human body, in order to obtain an effective reading from the reader, the minimum separation is 2 mm between the tag and the body. Combined, metal and human body (metal-zip wallet in a pocket) decrease the read range to an impractical distance. Separation between HF card and UHF card must be approximately with 4 non-RFID cards (credit card, ID).

We don't recommend an UHF sticker in a previously deployed HF card. It is necessary a separation between both tags. In accordance to the preferences of the personal, the best solution is to use a dual card that can works in UHF and HF. The second option is use a hanged UHF card for tracking and a HF card for the access control.

As a conclusion to the experiment, we suggest the following considerations to be taken into account in the implementation of a passive RFID localization system:

- Place the readers of the system in vertical position (horizontal reading) to improve the readings of tags.
- Guarantee a separation between tags and human or metallic bodies of at least 2 mm. It is advisable to attach a a non-metallic cover with the tag to abstract the user of these issues.
- Calibrate reader power depending of the precision desired.

References

1. Xiong, J., Seet, B.C., Symonds, J.: Human activity inference for ubiquitous rfid-based applications. In: Symposia and Workshops on Ubiquitous, Autonomic and Trusted Computing, pp. 304–309 (2009)
2. Bouet, M., Dos Santos, A.L.: Rfid tags: Positioning principles and localization techniques. In: 2008 1st IFIP Wireless Days, pp. 1–5 (2008)
3. Cangialosi, A., Monaly, J., Yang, S.: Leveraging rfid in hospitals: Patient life cycle and mobility perspectives. Communications Magazine 45(9), 18–23 (2007)
4. NextPoints, http://www.nextpoints.com/sectores.php?idioma=en
5. Inditar, http://www.inditar.com/control-acceso-rfid
6. Finkenzeller, K.: RFID Handbook: Fundamentals and Applications in Contactless Smart Cards and Identification, 2nd edn. John Wiley & Sons, Inc., New York (2003)
7. Recio, I., Moya, J.M., Araujo, Á., Vallejo, J.C., Malagón, P.: Analysis and design of an object tracking service for intelligent environments. In: Omatu, S., Rocha, M., Bravo, J., Riverola, F.F., Corchado, E., Bustillo, A., Corchado, J.M. (eds.) IWANN 2009. LNCS, vol. 5518, pp. 914–921. Springer, Heidelberg (2009)
8. Solic, P., Rozic, N., Ukic, N.: Roads: Rfid office application for document tracking over sip. In: Proceedings of the 17th International Conference on Software, Telecommunications and Computer Networks, SoftCOM 2009, pp. 95–100. IEEE Press, Piscataway (2009)
9. Zhang, Y., Amin, M.G.: Localization and tracking of passive RFID tags. Wireless Sensing and Processing (2006); Rao, Raghuveer M., Dianat, Sohail, A., Zoltowski, Michael, D. (eds.) Proceedings of the SPIE, vol. 6248, pp. 624809 (2006), Presented at the Society of Photo-Optical Instrumentation Engineers (SPIE) Conference (June 2006)
10. Wang, C., Wu, H., Tzeng, N.F.: Rfid-based 3-d positioning schemes. In: INFOCOM, pp. 1235–1243. IEEE, Los Alamitos (2007)
11. Bekkali, A., Sanson, H., Matsumoto, M.: Rfid indoor positioning based on probabilistic rfid map and kalman filtering. In: WiMob, p. 21. IEEE Computer Society, Los Alamitos (2007)
12. NXP, http://www.mifare.net/products/mifare-smartcard-ic-s/mifare-plus/
13. DailyRFID,
    http://www.rfid-in-china.com/2010-08-30/products_detail_2281.html

Emergency System for Elderly – A Computer Vision Based Approach

Rainer Planinc and Martin Kampel

Vienna University of Technology, Computer Vision Lab,
Favoritenstr. 9/183, A-1040 Vienna, Austria
{rainer.planinc,martin.kampel}@tuwien.ac.at
http://www.caa.tuwien.ac.at/cvl

Abstract. Elderly tend to forget or refuse wearing devices belonging to an emergency system (e.g. panic button). A vision based approach does not require any sensors to be worn by the elderly and is able to detect falls automatically. This paper gives an overview of my thesis, where different fall detection approaches are evaluated and combined. Furthermore, additional knowledge about the scene is incorporated to enhance the robustness of the system. To verify its feasibility, extensive tests under laboratory settings and real environments are conducted.

Keywords: ambient assisted living, fall detection, elderly, risk detection, autonomous system.

1 Introduction

Emergency systems for elderly contain at least one sensor (button or accelerometer), which has to be worn or pressed in case of emergency. These emergency call buttons are provided by care taker organizations having the main drawback that no information about an occurred incident prior the button press is available. Moreover, people have to wear these buttons which they tend to forget or even refuse. In case of an emergency and if elderly are able to press the button, they have to tell the operator, which kind of incident happened. If the elderly is not able to talk to the operator for any reason, there is no information about the type of incident at all. This causes false alarms as well as ambulance deployments, although there is no emergency situation at all. To ensure the detection of emergency situations where the elderly is not able to actively raise an alarm (e.g. due to the lost of consciousness), sensors acting autonomously are needed.

Autonomously acting sensors are used in the field of smart homes to fulfill core functions defined in [10]: the control of the system, emergency help, water and energy monitoring, automatic lighting, door surveillance, cooker safety, etc.. Due to various reasons summarized in [9], smart homes are not established yet. One of the reasons mentioned in [9] are costs: it is easier and less expensive to integrate smart home technology into new buildings than it is for already existing buildings. This results in the demand of a robust system, which can be integrated into existing buildings. Moreover, one of the outcome of the former

J. Bravo, R. Hervás, and V. Villarreal (Eds.): IWAAL 2011, LNCS 6693, pp. 79–83, 2011.

project MuBisA is that elderly accept technical assistance only if the system is not discernible for third persons. For these people, assistance means covert assistance in physical or intellectual impairment as long as possible, being hidden especially when it comes to visitors not belonging to the family or the innermost circle of friends. A small, low–key system would fulfill that demand.

Considering these facts, a computer vision approach is feasible as it is able to overcome the limitations of other sensor types [11]. Furthermore, not only falls can be detected but also other events where help is needed (e.g. fire, flooding,...). By the use of a vision based system the detection of emergency situations is done by software, meaning that this system is extendable as only the algorithms need to be extended or adopted. A wide variety of computer vision algorithms for different applications exist (e.g. [5,6,7,8]), but there is no "perfect" algorithm for detecting emergencies in elderly's homes yet.

As falls are considered to be a major risk for elderly, there has been done research on automatic fall detection [4]. Not only the fall itself but also the consequences of a fall are a great risk for elderly. [1] have shown that getting help quickly after a fall reduces the risk of death by over 80% and the risk of hospilization by 26%.

The rest of this document is structured as follows: Sect. 2 gives an overview over the State–of–the–Art. The methodology is shown in Sect. 3, an evaluation can be found in Sec. 4. Finally, a conclusion is presented in Sect. 5.

2   State–of–the–Art

In general there are two main approaches to detect falls – either elderly have to wear sensors (e.g. accelerometers, [3]) or falls are detected by computer vision systems (e.g. [5,6,7,8]). For our work, only the latter are of interest as we are not dealing with any kind of wearable sensors.

The general methodology of a fall detection systems is described in [4]. At first, people needs to be separated from the background. Therefore, motion detection and background subtraction is used. After the human is detected in the video, different kind of fall detection approaches are used. These approaches can be distinguished between 2D and 3D approaches. To be able to reconstruct a scene in 3D, a calibrated camera setup is needed.

When using a 2D approach, only limited information about the person is available. The shape of the person implies the orientation and thus can be used to distinguish whether a person is in an upright position or not. The bounding box aspect ratio (width to height ratio) to detect falls is used in [5]. If people are in an upright position, the ratio of the height to the width of the bounding box is bigger than one. If a fall occurs, the ratio rapidly changes to a value smaller than one. Another approach presented in [6] does not use the information of a bounding box but of an approximated ellipse. Falls are detected by analyzing the orientation of the ellipse.

Approaches making use of 3D information try to reconstruct humans from silhouettes gained by different camera views [7]. Hence, the human is represented by the use of voxels allowing to identify different states (upright, on–the–ground and in–between). Another approach presented in [8] uses 3D information to track the head of the person and to obtain its trajectory. Not only the head position but also the velocity of movement is taken as an indicator for falls as the velocity of movement during a fall is typically higher than during usual activities of daily living.

3   Methodology

Systems to detect falls using different approaches (e.g. 3D head tracking [8], aspect ratio of bounding box [5]) already exist. Hence, the use of these approaches and their results are evaluated. Based on this evaluation, improvements and combinations of feasible approaches are developed. Furthermore, additional knowledge of the scene is taken into account and is integrated to enhance the overall stability of the system. As the error rate of such systems should be low, not only the fall itself but also the whole environment has to be considered due to the similarities in movement between falls and other activities of daily living. Hence the structure of the scene needs to be taken into consideration, facilitating an overview and thus enabling decision making to be more robust.

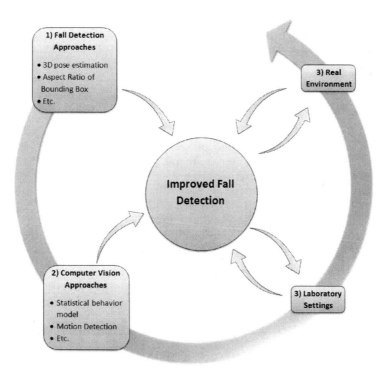

Fig. 1. Methodology

Due to the combination of different approaches, the system does not rely on one single approach only which increases the performance. To verify these assumptions, the algorithms are evaluated under laboratory settings as well as in real environments (i.e. elderly in their homes) comprehensively. Figure 1 shows an overview of the methodology: 1) different fall detection approaches are evaluated, 2) fall detection approaches are combined together with additional scene knowledge, 3) comprehensive evaluation and verification is done under a) laboratory settings and b) in real environments.

4   Evaluation

Our developed system is a specific solution for indoor environments. Thus it is able to handle challenges which can be typically found in indoor environments like illumination changes due to switching the lights on or off as well as movements without any information (e.g. the movement of curtains due to wind) which effects the motion detection. These factors need to be taken into account to develop a robust system. Therefore it is not sufficient to test the developed algorithms at laboratory settings, but also in real environments comprehensively.

The aim of our work is to ensure that critical situations like falls are detected while having a low false alarm rate. Hence, the developed algorithms need to be adopted to the use in elderly's homes. Currently no known system is able to detect all kinds of falls correctly as the movement during a fall can be mistaken with other activities of daily living (e.g. sitting down, lying on the bed, etc.). Within this work a robust method which is able to distinguish between activities of daily living and falls is developed. Therefore not only the development of one specific fall detection approach leads to success, but a combination of different fall detection approaches together with incorporated additional knowledge about the scene (e.g. a statistical behavior model introduced in [2]).

Figure 2 shows anonymized snapshots of the system. Since we use cameras within the homes of elderly, privacy and the protection of data is very important. To ensure the dignity of elderly, the system anonymizes the video stream automatically.

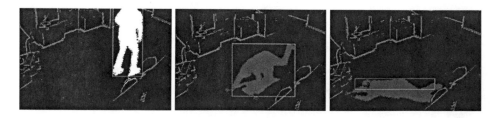

Fig. 2. Anonymized snapshots taken by the system

5 Conclusion

To be able to develop an efficient and robust vision based fall detection system, a combination of different approaches is feasible. The integration of other computer vision approaches like behavior models enhances the overall robustness of the system furthermore. Nonetheless, the system has to be evaluated within real settings as well. Only this ensures that all factors (e.g. moving curtains, rapidly changing light conditions, etc.) are considered.

References

1. Noury, N., Rumeau, P., Bourke, A.K., Laighin, G., Lundy, J.E.: A Proposal for the Classification and Evaluation of Fall Detectors. BioMedical Engineering and Research (IRBM) 29, 340–349 (2008)
2. Zweng, A., Zambanini, S., Kampel, M.: Introducing a Statistical Behavior Model into Camera-Based Fall Detection. In: Proc. of the 6th International Symposium on Visual Computing, Las Vegas, USA, pp. 163–172 (2010)
3. Lindemann, U., Hock, A., Stuber, M., Keck, W., Becker, C.: Evaluation of a fall detector based on accelerometers: A pilot study. Medical & Biological Engineering & Computing 43, 548–551 (2005)
4. Willems, J., Debard, G., Bonroy, B., Vanrumste, B., Goedem, T.: How to detect human fall in video? An overview. In: Proc. of the International Conference on Positioning and Context-Awareness, Antwerp (2009) (to be published)
5. Anderson, D., Keller, J.M., Skubic, M., Chen, X., He, Z.: Recognizing falls from silhouettes. In: Proc. of the 28th Annual International Conference on Engineering in Medicine and Biology Society (EMBS), New York, pp. 6388–6391 (2006)
6. Rougier, C., Meunier, J., St-Arnaud, A., Rousseau, J.: Fall Detection from Human Shape and Motion History Using Video Surveillance. In: Proc. of the 21st International Conference on Advanced Information Networking and Applications Workshops (AINAW), Niagara Falls, pp. 875–880 (2007)
7. Anderson, D., Luke, R.H., Keller, J.M., Skubic, M., Rantz, M., Aud, M.: Linguistic Summarization of Video for Fall Detection Using Voxel Person and Fuzzy Logic. Computer Vision and Image Understanding 113, 80–89 (2009)
8. Rougier, C., Meunier, J., St-Arnaud, A., Rousseau, J.: Monocular 3D head tracking to detect falls of elderly people. In: Proc. of the 28th Annual International Conference on Engineering in Medicine and Biology Society (EMBS), New York, pp. 6384–6387 (2006)
9. Aldrich, F.: Smart Homes: Past, Present and Future. In: Harper, R. (ed.) Inside the Smart Home, pp. 17–39. Springer, London (2003)
10. Fisk, M.J.: The implication of smart home technologies. In: Peace, S.M., Holland, C. (eds.) Inclusive housing in an ageing society: innovative approaches, pp. 101–124. Policy Press, Bristol (2001)
11. Mihailidis, A., Carmichael, B., Boger, J.: The Use of Computer Vision in an Intelligent Environment to Support Aging-in-Place, Safety, and Independence in the Home. IEEE Transactions on Information Technology in Biomedicine 3, 238–247 (2004)

Communication Architecture for Tracking and Interoperable Services at Hospitals: A Real Deployment Experience

Augusto Morales, Tomás Robles, Ramón Alcarria, and David Alonso

Technical University of Madrid, Avenida Complutense. 30,
28040 Madrid, Spain
{amorales,trobles,ralcarria}@dit.upm.es
david.alonso.abarca@alumnos.upm.es

Abstract. Any new hospital communication architecture has to support existing services, but at the same time new added features should not affect normal tasks. This article deals with issues regarding old and new systems' interoperability, as well as the effect the human factor has in a deployed architecture. It also presents valuable information, which is a product of a real scenario. Tracking services are also tested in order to monitor and administer several medical resources.

Keywords: RFID, OSGi, SIP, Tracking, real-deployment.

1 Introduction

Medical environments are dynamic and this affects the way standard processes are accomplished. In recent years, new ideas related to drug tracking, smart medical services, and patient monitoring have been transformed into successful systems. In addition, there are technologies such as: Radio Frequency Identification (RFID)[1], Open Service Gateway Initiative (OSGi)[2], Session Initiation Protocol (SIP)[3] that have certainly demonstrated [4][5][6] through different mechanisms that they can enrich medical environments by extending the capabilities to many devices. As a result, there are new trends for applying alternative technologies in order to address hospital communication issues to support future medical services.

Medical environments have different requirements that restrict the way new technology, architecture, protocol or system can be integrated into an existing communication model. Therefore, there are some problems regarding interaction between the medical staff and the technology itself. This interdisciplinary fact affects the way AAL is provided to patients or handicapped people whom need support in their own house or in hospitals.

This paper is based on a previously proposed architecture [7], where we considered some problems regarding sensors and medical services as well as their integration with legacy hospital networks and processes. This architecture has an open-service model based on OSGi, so new medical services can be deployed without modifying other running applications. In this way, the architecture could be seen as the core of future characteristics provided by an AAL platform.

J. Bravo, R. Hervás, and V. Villarreal (Eds.): IWAAL 2011, LNCS 6693, pp. 84–91, 2011.
© Springer-Verlag Berlin Heidelberg 2011

This paper is focused on the deployment issues the CARDINEA project [8] consortium had to overcome in order to integrate existing medical systems with new features, sensors and services. It also proposes alternatives to address hospital requirements such as: drugs, equipment and medical staff tracking. We describe our fully-operational prototype which carried out real medical data and processes. On the other hand, there are several alternatives for analyzing valid system integrations; though we limit our scope to the deployment itself and the challenges we have to deal to, such as: physical location, resource availability and staff cooperation.

1.1 Challenges

Nowadays medical environments have challenges in several areas. One of them is tracking. If we analyze specific scenarios, for example one floor specialized in intern medicine; we conclude that tracking can be applied to many things such as: expensive drugs, medical equipment, nursing and so on.

Actually, some hospitals keep manual tracking of the drugs, since they are received until they are administered to patients. This manual process takes time and is susceptible to human error [10]. Thus, drug tracking has a direct impact on the overall efficiency of a hospital's pharmacy, as well as it also prevents to lose costly or limited drugs.

Tracking of medical devices involves an important point of the whole hospital process. In addition, it inherits the same deficiencies, if manual processing is in operation. Expensive devices can be lost, stolen or be inadequately used. Nevertheless, automatic tracking overcomes them, as well as the hospital can optimize its resources when unforeseen events occur.

Staff tracking is particularly challenging because it involves humans. It is necessary in critical cases when emergencies occur or when patients need continuous monitoring. It has been proven that medical errors can be minimized [11] by using communication systems, so medical staff monitoring can help to administer drugs in the correct way, amount and time. On the other hand, medical staff tracking is difficult because it involves other human aspects such as: privacy and trust.

Another challenge is concerning patients and their **vital constant monitoring.** Hospitals have systems in order to monitor and send alarms to medical staff when special situations occur. Otherwise, some of those systems are proprietary, so the integration among Hospital Information Systems (HIS) may be complicated. Adding the new features cannot modify or affect existing medical services, process, systems or data.

It is not easy to integrate a single hospital scenario with current and new systems. Integration of technologies is indeed challenging. It includes networks, bio-sensors, medical devices, and specialized database such as HIS. However, another challenge concerns **humans and their willingness** to use new processes, or systems. Thus, integration with health personnel and technical supporting people requires training, as well as direct feedback from them, since there are the people that will adopt the technology. Furthermore, on-site testing is crucial for any successful system and the perception medical staff will experience.

Since our architecture is based on **integration between different medical systems,** and involves human interaction, we have implemented the prototype in the

Hospital de Terrassa, Catalunya, Spain. This functional prototype has been integrated with existing hospital systems, so real medical staff has interacted with it.

In the next section we briefly explain the top level architecture for the prototype. Following that we describe the deployment process, requirements and other considerations for the testing scenario. The next section describes results and problems addressed, and finally we finish with a discussion and lessons learned.

2 Architecture

The architecture proposed in the CARDINEA project integrates different modules and technologies. The architecture is based on hierarchical levels and supports different logical or physical areas.

Figure number 1 shows the modules developed and how all of them are integrated in the same architecture with OSGi as the main platform. The modules involved [7] are Open Context Platform (OCP) [9], Enterprise Service Beans (ESB), SIP, Mirth and RFID. The OCP module stores information regarding sensors, patients, staff, drugs, as well as the location data of them. Next, it organizes these data into a defined ontology. The ESB module registers the information received from the Hospital Information System (HIS) into the OCP context. This information is used to create the different entities needed in the ontology for storing all the biomedical data for further analyzing. The SIP module negotiates the communication channels taking into consideration the biomedical information and the current network conditions. The RFID module controls the antennas and RFID readers intended for the detection of the location. Finally, the Mirth module receives parameters from the SIP session and sends/receives the Health Level 7 (HL7) [12] compliant data by using the proper quality of service values.

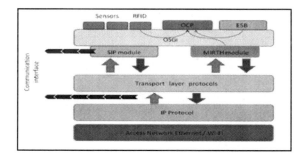

Fig. 1. Central Server Topology Layers

3 From Architecture to Implementation

In any real deployment, the architecture may be limited by the existing physical and technological resources of the scenario. On the other hand, the architecture has to be adaptable without modifying its high level functions and purpose. As we mentioned before, our prototype was test-driven in a real hospital scenario which had many constrains.

The physical element affects many technological factors such as: the antenna power for reading RFID tags, the available Bluetooth range and Wi-Fi availability. In this case, a wall's thickness and its material can affect the overall system performance. Alternatively, wired connectivity can be used to ensure good quality network communication, but it can be very invasive for testing a temporary system. Furthermore, a successful architecture deployment needs a balance between functionality, and non-invasive techniques. This last characteristic is undeniably important for medical and other AAL environments, which cannot be frequently modified.

In our deployment there were several wireless devices such as: Health Station, RFID readers and sensors that made use of wireless connectivity. It is clear that these devices are designed to avoid interferences and comply with many safety regulations. Despite this, we had to deal with some packet lost, Bluetooth interference, and in some cases, medical staff complaints. Thus, using wireless devices in medical environments have clear advantages and disadvantages.

The architecture defined several hierarchical levels with the aim of maintaining the separation between different hospital floors. This design allows continuing the communication system running even if one of the network devices fails. The physical and technological resources available in the Hospital did not permit the deployment of the complete architecture based on different roles and servers. As a solution, we unified the Intermediate Server with the Central Server into one single component. This change was suitable because the logical modules are OSGi bundles and can be seamless executed in the same server. In this case, the architecture's design based on the OSGi's flexibility allowed us an adaptable and fast deployment.

The prototype was deployed by implementing different software elements of the architecture. Each software element, and its functionality, was executed by an OSGi bundle. As we previously mentioned, the OSGi platform allows a quick integration. Even thought, in a real deployment which involves several developers and software components, a successful system requires time indeed. Thus, even when OSGi has methods for publishing bundles and their functionalities, via standardized interfaces, data format and data exchange are still issues in real scenarios.

3.1 Deployed Architecture and Workflow

Finally the architecture has suffered some changes due to the fact that it had to be implemented in a real test scenario. The scenario featured some installation restrictions that were motivated by the placement of equipment and the possibility of disturbing the patients and the health personnel.

On the other hand, we had to make topology changes because of the available hospital resources. Figure 2 shows the topology of the test scenario. In the first step, the health stations collect (1) all the medical information from the biomedical sensors. Next, they send (2) the medical data to the HIS, which is a legacy communication system used by the hospital and stores all the patient records. This HIS also execute data coding in HL7 format, establishes the correct data session and send (3) HL7 data to the Central server. Meanwhile, the RFID sub-system, which is totally independent of other modules, detects the RFID tags from nurses, drugs, patients and sensors, so it can send (4) these events to the Central Server.

The test scenario achieves external communication with the HIS using a 3G router. By doing this, it did not interfere with the other systems installed and complied with hospital's regulations. All the information collected in the Central Server is processed and organized in a previously defined ontology by the OCP module, which also generates a context model. Therefore, any other module in the OSGi platform could later consume this information.

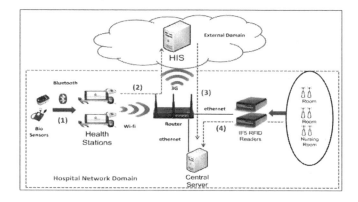

Fig. 2. Deployed system and workflow

3.2 Hospital Deployment

The prototype has been test-driven using the Open Source FUSE ESB [13] as the OSGi Framework for the Central server. It also ran Ubuntu 10.04 with Java SDK 1.6 and 1GB RAM. The Health Stations ran Windows XP Embedded version with 1GB RAM. The RFID readers were the Intermec IF5 [14] model, running an embedded version of Linux OS and JADE [15] 3.7.0 version as the OSGi framework.

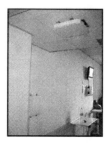
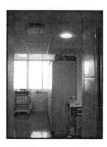
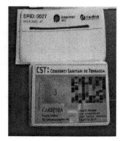

Fig. 3. Patient Room   **Fig. 4.** Nurse station   **Fig. 5.** RFID Tags

As we previously stated, the whole prototype was located in the Terrassa Hospital's fifth floor. This floor specializes in intern medicine. There were three places with RFID passage arches: two patient rooms and one nursing room. Each arch had two antennas to guarantee the reading of RFID tags. The RFID readers, which processed tags and managed antenna reception power, were located on the top of the ceiling. There was

Ethernet communication from the readers to the Central server, as well as Wi-Fi link as a backup up channel. The Central server was placed in the nurse station.

The Health Station, depicted in figure 6, was attached to the nursing trolley, as well as the glucometer, pulsimeter and tensiometer sensors. These devices sent their monitored vital constants to the Health Station, via Bluetooth connection. Then, the Health Station sent these data to the HIS using its Wi-Fi connection.

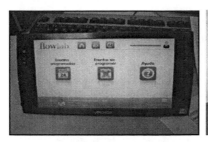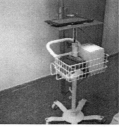

Fig. 6. Health Station and nursing trolley

The nursing trolley had a RFID tag which allowed the system to detect the time when vital constants were registered for data processing. The nurses also carried the same sort of RFID tag in their pockets for a similar purpose. Location was also recorded by monitoring patients and nurses RFID tags. At the beginning of the testing-time, the system noticed a low rate of RFID tag events because of the hospital's physical characteristics, including the metallic nursing trolley employed. As a solution the RFID working frequency was adjusted between 865 and 868 MHz and the reader output power was also set to the maximum available rate (30.0 dBm). These changes significantly improved the system performance. With the proper tuning, the tracking system preliminary results showed that during nine testing days the activity average rate for nurses and trolleys was 12.66 RFID location events per day. The nurse station had 8.77 events and the rooms 3.89. These first results matched with the periodic nurses rounds in the hospital. Gathered data analyzing time has not finished yet. However, at this time, we did extract useful information from health personnel surveys. The system did not affect regular medical task, so medical staff could perfectly continue working with patients which was especially important for the prototype success.

4   Discussion

Any evolution from current to future stages in any hospital systems is difficult and risky, especially when it involves a drastic change. Taking this into consideration, we have realized that experimenting with real systems, process and humans is necessary for successful hospital architectures and general AAL environments.

There are many issues regarding deploying new medical systems into real scenarios. One of them is *interoperability of systems*. Our OSGi based architecture was mainly focused on this fact. Nevertheless, for real working scenarios, it is especially difficult to troubleshot problems when different software components have to interoperate. In addition, this issue can be even worse when remote access support is not enough, because on-site testing can be difficult and sometimes frustrating for patients, medical staff and so on. Therefore, previous and extensive system testing is a mandatory requirement for any medical deployment,

Cooperation and feedback with medical staff and patients are indispensable. Our architecture involved a human component by suggesting to medical staff to always carry a RFID tag in their pockets. In this way, this new sort of request has to be adapted to their comfort and cannot affect their daily tasks. Thus, adding touch screen technologies seems to be less invasive, improves the system usability, and the willingness to continue testing new systems.

Since a prototype cannot affect a Hospital, its normal processes and communication systems, *efficient physical deploying* is a requirement. Our prototype involved bothersome infrastructural changes for the RFID equipment installation. However, once the antennas were in their position, our architecture allowed us to change settings such as: antenna power, antennas covering and so on, in order to adapt the prototype. As a result, *software flexibility* allowed us to avoid physical alterations. Evidently *Privacy* was also taken into consideration. Our experiences in this development, via surveys, suggest to us that tracking, which involves privacy aspects, is not totally-accepted by health personnel. As a result, it was necessary to correctly explain and define the purpose of the collected data. Thus, in our testing system the location information was only employed to obtain statistical data.

4.1 Lessons Learned

As we expected, the testing scenario had undeniably provided us valuable information. Our data analysis, which will provide us with statistical results, has not been finalized yet, but we have learned lessons regarding this architecture and its capabilities. Taking all the deployment challenges into consideration, we first requested, to the Hospital's administration, two sorts of phases for our testing scenario. The first phase was focused on system tuning, and the second phase for data collecting. However, our short period of two week was not enough because the testing phase was also limited by human factors such as medical staff and patients' availability. Therefore, these types of random factors have to be taken in account when testing time is restricted to the internal hospital policy.

The original architecture envisaged service creation from specialized developers. On the other hand, the medical staff's surveys demonstrated that creating basic and simple services will be one of the best advantages for future hospitals and AAL environments. Thus, personal devices such as: mobile phones or PDA could have mechanisms for creating medical services that interact with HIS or similar hospital systems. In addition, staff location and alarms could be integrated as key service features. Since medical staff's tracking is still an uncompleted feature in our system, a future architecture will have to include location policy modules.

Our prototype made use of several wireless technologies for communicating devices. However, for future deployments it would be positive to support other technologies such as 6LowPAN or Zigbee. This attribute, in conjunction with Wi-Fi, will extend the monitoring capabilities and ensure the control of data flow in case of failure or unforeseen situations.

Alternatively, the participation and interaction of the medical staff was also difficult, for two main reasons. At the beginning, the prototype setup time seemed to be frustrating for them, but it was almost an unavoidable fact. Additionally, the natural human mistrust of new technology affected the expected first feedbacks. Nevertheless, after the training days, medical staff could adopt the new procedures, and finally noticed system features including the round time optimization achieved by using wireless communication. This fact was directly reflected in having more availability to take care of patients.

To summarize, our deployment experience provides practical feedback in order to adapt and improve future communication architectures. Since testing is one of the methods to accomplish upcoming integration of health services, this paper has identified challenges in current scenarios, as well as analyzing and proposing suitable solutions.

Acknowledgement

This work is supported by the Ministry of Industry, Tourism and Commerce of Spain, through "Avanza I+D Subprogram" and Project CARDINEA number TSI-020302-2009-43, and TIN T2C2 (TIN2008-06739-C04-03).

References

[1] Association of Automatic identification and Mobility, http://www.rfid.org (accessed on January 2011)
[2] OSGi Alliance Website, http://www.osgi.org (accessed on January 2011)
[3] Rosenberg, J., Schulzrinne, H., Camarillo, G., Johnston, A., Peterson, J., Sparks, R., Handley, M., Schooler, E.: SIP: Session Initiation Protocol. Internet Engineering Task Force, RFC 3261 (June 2002)
[4] Lopez, P.P., Orfila, A., Mitrokotsa, A., van der Lubbe, J.C.A.: A comprehensive RFID solution to enhance inpatient medication safety. International Journal of Medical Informatics (2010)
[5] Lin, W.-W., Sheng, Y.H.: Using OSGi UPnP and Zigbee to provide a wireless ubiquitous home healthcare environment. In: The Second International Conference on Mobile Ubiquitous Computing, Systems, Services and Technologies (2008)
[6] Sadat, A., Sorwar, G., Chowdhury, M.U.: Session Initiation Protocol (SIP) based Event Notification System Architecture for Telemedicine Applications. In: Proceedings of the 5th IEEE/ACIS International Conference on Computer and Information Science (2006)
[7] Morales, A., Valladares, T.R., Alcarria, R., Alonso, D., Platas, S.: Communication Architecture for Smart Service in Hospital Environments. In: Proceedings of Workshop of Ambient Assisted Living, IWAAL 2010, Valencia, Spain, pp. 61–68 (2010)
[8] Cardinea Project Homepage, http://cardinea.grupogesfor.com (accessed on March 2011)
[9] Open Context Platform OCP2, http://ants-webs.inf.um.es/ocp2 (accessed on March 2011)
[10] Hughes, R.G., Ortiz, E.: Medication errors: why they happen, and how they can be prevented. American Journal of Nursing 105, 14–24 (2005)
[11] Benjamin, D.M.: Reducing medication errors and increasing patient safety: case studies in clinical pharmacology. Journal of Clinical Pharmacology 43, 768–783 (2003)
[12] HL7 Health Level Seven International, http://www.hl7.org (accessed on January 2011)
[13] Fuse Source Open source SOA, http://www.fusesource.com (accessed on January 2011)
[14] Intermec Website, http://www.intermec.com (accessed on January 2011)
[15] Java Agent Development Framework, http://jade.tilab.com (accessed on January 2011)

Live Interactive Frame Technology Alleviating Children Stress and Isolation during Hospitalization

Pablo Antón, Antonio Maña, Antonio Muñoz, and Hristo Koshutanski

Escuela Técnica Superior de Ingeniería Informtica
Universidad de Málaga
{panton,amg,amunoz,hristo}@lcc.uma.es

Abstract. Children that spend long periods in hospitals suffer different negative effects that affect their emotional and psychological development including sleep disorders, stress, and degradation of school performance. A common reason behind these effects is related to breaking of normal relationships and lack of contacts with the daily environments (family, friends, school, etc.). In this paper we describe a system called Live Interactive Frame (LIFE), developed in DESEOS research project, to address this situation. The LIFE system provides children with live interactive visual contact of their school activities during hospitalization with the goal of reducing the stress and feeling of isolation.

1 Introduction

Ambient Intelligence (AmI) is a paradigm where Information Technology is applied to build networks of devices and services that are dynamically connected and collaborate to help people in different activities. These digital environments are aware of the presence of people, and can react and adapt to their necessities, habits, and movements [8]. Ambient Assisting Living (AAL) systems are designed to assist people with disabilities or health problems with the main goal of extending the period of time in which they live independently in their daily environment. Despite of the fact that this technology was initially designed to be applied to elderly and handicapped people [19,7], today more and more scenarios for AAL are being developed.

In this paper we present an application of AmI technologies to develop an AAL system helping children that undergo long-term hospitalization periods, where this technology can offer interesting advantages. Children that have to spend long periods in hospitals suffer different negative effects that affect their emotional and psychological development and their family life [14,17]. Some of the effects that have been studied and focus of our research are:

1. *Sleep disorders.* The experience of the medical and psychological team of DESEOS has revealed that even in cases of mild diseases, the children that stay in hospitals suffer sleep disorders that tend to be transitory, but that can have negative effects in the children's and their relatives' lives.

J. Bravo, R. Hervás, and V. Villarreal (Eds.): IWAAL 2011, LNCS 6693, pp. 92–100, 2011.

2. *Stress.* Stress is one of the most common effects of the stay in hospitals, both in children and their parents [2]. Studies reveal that this stress is caused to a great extent by isolation and lack of contact with their daily environments.

3. *Consequences on school performance.* This effect is not only caused by sickness, which undoubtedly has a negative influence on the children' education [18], but again has a strong relation with the lack of human contact and affection [1]. Several studies show that this happens even in cases in which the disease or sickness did not have a direct influence on the capabilities and abilities for studying of the child.

A common reason behind these effects seems to be related with the breaking of normal relationships and lack of contact with the daily environments (family, friends, school, etc.). In psychology, the effects of the contact (or lack thereof) with others are related to the concept of 'attachment'. By definition, attachment describes *"the state and quality of an individual's emotional ties to another"* [4]. Attachment theory was conceived by British psychiatrist and psychoanalyst John Bowlby. According to him, the *"observation of how a very young child behaves towards his mother, both in her presence and especially in her absence, can contribute greatly to our understanding of personality development"* [5].

Many different studies have shown the importance of the attachment between children and parents and also with the social groups they belong to, and have emphasized the role of visual contact and interactivity as solid basis for attachment. Attachment relationships have a *"direct effect on the development of the domains of mental functioning that serve as our conceptual anchor points; memory, narrative function, representations, and state of mind"* [21]. In fact, attachment relationships may serve to create the central foundation from which the mind develops [15].

Maintaining attachment bonds is especially important in stressful situations, like the ones we are addressing in DESEOS. In reference [6] we read *"The infant and young child seeks closeness, especially to the mother, when he experiences anxiety. This may occur when, for example, he is separated from his mother, encounters threatening unfamiliar situations or strange persons, experiences physical pain, or feels overwhelmed by his fantasies, as in nightmares"*. Not surprisingly, the parent-child relationship is not the only one that affects the development of the child. Bruce D. Perry states: *"There is no more specific 'biological' determinant than a relationship. Human beings evolved as social animals and the majority of biology of the brain is dedicated to mediating the complex interactions required to keep small, naked, weak, individual humans alive by being part of a larger biological whole -the family, the clan-"* [20].

It is widely recognized that visual contact and facial expressions provide important social and emotional information. Indeed, visual contact is arguably the most important form of non-verbal communication [16]. With regards to the role of visual contact in this attachment process Karl H. Brisch states: *"This search for closeness may be accompanied by visual contact with the mother or, especially, by seeking close bodily contact with her"* [6]. Furthermore, recent studies suggest that eye contact has a positive impact on the retention and recall of information and may promote more efficient learning [9]. More recently, the importance of visual contact in remote communication has been determined [10].

The main target of the DESEOS project is the development and application of secure technologies for Ambient Assisted Living (AAL) systems to increase the quality of life of health cared children by developing novel devices and applications to enhance the contact with the different daily environments. With this goal, and based on the previous studies about the importance of visual contact and interactivity in the perception of closeness and immersion into the quotidian social relationships, we have developed a novel AAL system, called LIFE (Live Interactive FramE), providing an immersive interactive view of two separate physical spaces, used to help children maintain the contact with their school and to participate in classroom activities while being hospitalized. We present the technologies, devices, and software architecture realizing LIFE. One important goal of DESEOS is to develop devices that can be easily and inexpensively built and integrated into existing systems. The paper also presents the main LIFE use case and an evaluation methodology allowing validation of the effectiveness of the technology in reducing the stress and feeling of isolation.

2 LIFE Application Scenario

The main objective of DESEOS is to build an AAL environment to improve quality of life for hospitalized children, both during the hospitalization period and during the post-hospitalization time. In order to achieve this objective the research and development in DESEOS is guided by several selected scenarios. In this section we present one of these scenarios in order to illustrate the kind of situations and systems that DESEOS deal with. The scenario focuses on the provision of means to reduce the problems caused by long-term hospitalization of children and involves two spaces (physical environments): Hospitals where children are hospitalized and Schools where the hospitalized children' classmates and teachers are. In the scenario we consider several roles depending on the actors that interact (parents, teachers, doctors, etc) and the space where the activity is developed (hospital, classroom, home, etc). Our general goal in this scenario is to make the hospitalized child be able to continue attending school in his own class. Although all hospitals have a school where children can continue their education, we believe that the most important aspect that the child loses is not the education (lectures, tuition and exercises) but the human contact and the integration in the group. Several subgoals guided us to build our scenario:

- *Visual contact.* Eyesight is one of the main senses in human communication and interaction. Providing technical means for maintaining visual contact in the most natural way so that the child feels that he is attending his normal class is therefore very important. For this purpose we provide a special type of video streaming service that we call "Live Interactive Frame (LIFE)" because it acts like a window changing the part of the classroom displayed depending on the position and viewing angle of the hospitalized child.

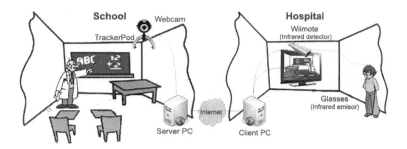

Fig. 1. LIFE Application Scenario

- *Auditory contact.* Another essential aspect in the communication is the auditory contact. It complements the visual contact helping the child getting integrated in his classroom as any other classmate. This is achieved integrating different microphones that are mixed depending on the relative position of the child and the Live Interactive Frame (LIFE).
- *Medical and school information.* In every situation there is certain information related with the hospitalized kid that is used by different actors. The level of access and the specific information that is made accessible is determined dynamically depending on the situation, the context and the actor.

We consider the following elements in each space: (i) A set of devices which form a local AmI environment (TV screens, webcams, microphones, electronic backboards, etc.), (ii) Information systems of particular domain (databases, servers, etc.), and (iii) A set of people who play different roles.

Figure 1 illustrates the elements in each of the spaces of the scenario. These elements are used to fulfil the above-mentioned goals. For instance, movable webcams and TV screens are used for achieving a satisfactory level of visual contact by implementing not only the LIFE application but also other uses like the replication of the classroom blackboard in the hospital room. To increase the feeling of natural interaction we use an accurate positioning system for the viewer (the hospitalized child) so that we can simulate the sensation of looking through a window by using camera movement and zooming. The positioning system uses a bluetooth infrared camera. For economy reasons we use a Nintendo Wii console remote for this purpose [13]. All devices shown in the figure have a role in order to make possible the interaction and the contact between hospitalized children and their schools. However, due to the nature of the managed information (medical, scholar, video, etc), some security issues arise which are addressed in [3].

LIFE Immersion View Effect. LIFE enables users to use a monitor (computer peripheral monitor) as a real world window giving the augmented impression of remote contact. This impression is achieved by means of sensing the user situation and movements to show the remote image according to these parameters. Transparently to user movements the motorized camera is rolled to provides the real world window impression. Figure 2 shows the virtual effect achieved. The

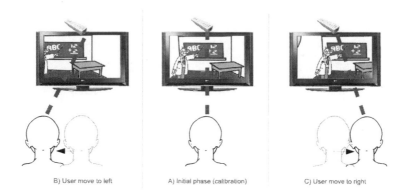

Fig. 2. LIFE Immersion View Effect

immersion view effect is the main aspect of DESEOS LIFE application providing the real psychological effect on hospitalized children.

3   LIFE Software Architecture

A general overview of the DESEOS LIFE architecture is illustrated in Figure 3. LIFE application uses a client-server model that establishes bidirectional communications between hospital and school realms. The WiiUseJ[1] library is used on the client side to access the Wiimote (remote control of the Wii system). The WiiUse dynamic access library connects the WiiUseJ layer and the bluetooth stack. The server-side architecture makes use of the functionality provided by the library Xuggler[2] used to capture video streaming from a webcam or an IP camera, changing encoding format, frames modification, and so on. This server is in charge of processing video streaming and performing Trackerpot[3] device rolling that adds pan and tilt (PTZ) properties to a video device. Tracketpot has an associated HTTP server in charge of accepting, processing and performing rolling on the physical device.

LIFE application provides bidirectional (client-server) communications by establishing two separate connections. When the server is started, a control socket is opened on a predefined port so that the server is waiting for a connection request. Once the connection is established on this socket some control parameters are set. The server captures the video streaming (of school realm webcam) using the functionality provided by Xuggler and streams the video out to the client (school realm) application using the RTP protocol. We note that the control connection is kept alive in order to receive the tilt, pan, zoom information coming from head tracking and send this information to the Trackerpot.

---

[1] http://code.google.com/p/wiiusej
[2] http://www.xuggle.com/xuggler
[3] http://www.trackercam.com/TCamWeb

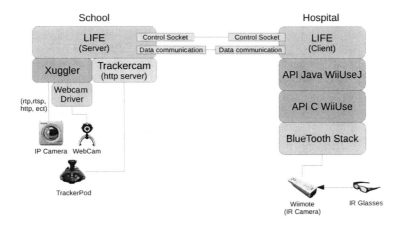

Fig. 3. LIFE Software Architecture

The head tracking on a client-side is implemented by using infrared wiimote sensor which locates user position by taking user infrared sunglasses as a reference point. The WiiUseJ library functionality is used to process input information from the wiimote sensor. The LIFE application decides how to transform video streaming frames to simulate the real movement and how much tilt, pan, and zoom is necessary to apply. Figure 4 shows the relation between the head position with the tilt, pan and zoom parameters.

Basically, we make use of trigonometry to calculate the ratio between user head position and the angles PTZ. The figure shows all directly related angles with the screen, user previous position and user current position. In the bottom right part of the figure we also show the functions used to calculate x, y and z values, known thanks to the wiimote use.

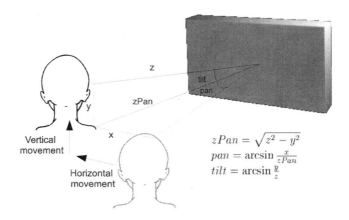

$$zPan = \sqrt{z^2 - y^2}$$
$$pan = \arcsin \frac{x}{zPan}$$
$$tilt = \arcsin \frac{y}{z}$$

Fig. 4. LIFE Tilt-Pan Calculation

4   Methodology Evaluation on Effectiveness of LIFE

An important part of LIFE technology is performing evaluation of its real psychological effect on reducing stress and isolation of hospitalized children. For this propose it has been defined a methodology of how to achieve evaluation on the effectiveness of the technology.

The objective of the methodology is to validate the pilot prototype of LIFE in collaboration with psychologies, teachers and doctors. The evaluation is planned to cover 30 school-age hospitalized children selected from the pediatrics unit at the Hospital Clínico Universitario de Granada[4]. The selection criteria is rather generic where the consensus of the parents and the child are required, as well as, acceptable conditions of the child for use of LIFE technology.

The evaluation follows these steps for every selected child:

1. Actigraphs start recording children information 72 prior to the evaluation of LIFE.
2. Questionnaires STAIC [22] and CDS [12] set control data of stress and anxiety levels of the child.
3. LIFE technology is used for a predefined period of time (e.g. a week). The time of use of LIFE is gradually incremented until it allows the child to follow classes in school. This papameter is defined in accordance to the actual school program and the doctors at the hospital.
4. Use an actigraph for 72 hours after the child has used the LIFE application to analyse the sleep-wake rhythms of the child and its motional conditions based on the data of steps 1 and 4.
5. Complete again the STAIC and CDS questionnaires after using LIFE to analyse the child stress and anxiety levels LIFE has induced.
6. Parents, teachers, family and doctors will complete a specific questionnaire evaluating level of satisfaction and acceptance of LIFE.

5   Related Work

A Virtual Window system [11] uses head movements in the viewer location to control camera movement in a remote location. The result is that viewers perceive that they are in front of a window allowing exploration of remote scenes rather than a flat screen showing moving pictures. This idea constitutes the starting point of our work.

Chung Lee [13] uses the infrared camera in the Wii remote and a head mounted sensor bar (two IR LEDs) to accurately track the location of user head and render view dependent images on the screen. This effectively transforms a display into a portal to a virtual environment. The display properly reacts to head and body movement as if it were a real window creating a realistic illusion of depth and space.

---

[4] http://www.juntadeandalucia.es/servicioandaluzdesalud/hsc/

6 Conclusion and Future Work

We have presented a novel AAL application, called LIFE, applying AmI technologies to increase the quality of life of health-cared children. The LIFE application scenario provides immersive interactive view of school activities taking place during children hospitalization. We have presented the technologies, devices, and software architecture underlying LIFE. We have also presented a LIFE use case evaluation and its related methodology to verify the effectiveness of the technology in reducing the stress and feeling of isolation.

Current prototype implementation allows unidirectional video streaming. A future work is to enable bidirectional (a second) video streaming channel of classmates seeing hospitalized kid. This is an important aspect from a psychological point of view of allowing hospitalized kids having visual feedback from their classmates in school. However, privacy issues are to be considered allowing the hospitalized children to disable the second video channel when they do not want to be seen in this way.

Another direction of future work is related to the performance of LIFE technology, as children might feel uncomfortable using the system if its reaction time is not small enough. Slow or inaccurate reaction of the system might lead to motion sickness. The evaluation results will help us determine these problems along with possible solutions based on calibration. However, we plan to provide a calibration setting where the system reaction time will be adjusted to fit the environment conditions and the user current emotional state.

Acknowledgements

This work is supported by the project **DESEOS** (TIC-4257, **D**ispositivos **E**lectrónicos **S**eguros para la **E**ducación, **O**cio y **S**ocialización) funded by the government of Andalucía (Spain).

References

1. Aguilar Cordero, M.J.: Influencia de la institucionalización y distintos modelos de acogida sobre el crecimiento, el desarrollo y el comportamiento en el síndrome de carencia afectiva en el niño. PhD thesis, Universidad de Granada (1995)
2. Aguilar Cordero, M.J., Galdó Muñoz, G., Muñoz Hoyos, A., Molina Carballo, A., Vallejo Bolaños, E., Ruiz Cosano, C., Valenzuela Ruiz, A.: Valoració del nivel de ansiedad estado/rasgo en niños institucionalizados. In: IV Congreso Estatal Infancia Maltratada (1995)
3. Antón, P., Muñoz, A., Maña, A., Koshutanski, H.: Security-enhanced ambient assisted living supporting school activities during hospitalisation. Journal of Ambient Intelligence and Humanized Computing, 1–16 (2010), doi:10.1007/s12652-010-0039-6
4. Becker-Weidman, A.: Dyadic Developmental Psychotherapy: The Theory. In: Creating capacity for attachment: Dyadic Developmental Psychotherapy in the treatment of trauma-attachment disorders, pp. 7–43. Wood 'N' Barnes (2005)

5. Bowlby, J.: Attachment and loss, 2nd edn. Attachment, vol. 1. Basic Books, New York (1982)
6. Brisch, K.H.: Treating Attachment Disorders From Theory to Therapy. The Guilford Press, New York (2002)
7. Corchado, J.M., Bajo, J., Abraham, A.: Gerami: Improving healthcare delivery in geriatric residences. IEEE Intelligent Systems 23(2), 19–25 (2008)
8. de Ruyter, B., Pelgrim, E.: Ambient assisted-living research in carelab. Interactions 14(4), 30 (2007)
9. Estrada, C.A., Patel, S.R., Talente, G., Kraemer, S.: The 10-minute oral presentation: what should i focus on? American Journal of the Medical Sciences 329, 306–309 (2005)
10. Fullwood, C., Doherty-Sneddon, G.: Effect of gazing at the camera during a video link on recall. Applied Ergonomics 37(2), 167–175 (2006)
11. Gaver, W.W., Smets, G., Overbeeke, K.: A Virtual Window on Media Space. In: CHI, pp. 257–264 (1995)
12. Lang, M., Tisher, M.: Children's Depression Scale (CDS). Australian Council for Educational Research
13. Lee, J.C.: Hacking the Nintendo Wii Remote. IEEE Pervasive Computing 7(3), 39–45 (2008)
14. Lockin, M.: The redefinition of failure to thrive from a case study perspective. Pediatric Nursing 31(6), 474–479 (2005)
15. McConahay, J.: Dyadic developmental psychotherapy: An exploration of attachment research and a look at a promising approach for treatment of attachment disorders. Master's thesis, Winona State University (2007)
16. Mehrabian, A.: Nonverbal Communication. Walter De Gruyter Inc., Berlin (1972)
17. Muñoz Hoyos, A.: Influencia de la institucionalización sobre el crecimiento, desarrollo y comportamiento en el niño. Part of the course: Principales problemas sociales en la infancia. Educación y cuidados. Escuela Universitaria de Ciencias de la Salud. Granada (1996)
18. Muñoz Hoyos, A.: Problemática del niño institucionalizado. Part of the Course: Pediatría Social. Universidad de Sevilla. Facultad de Medicina. Departamento de Pediatra, Sevilla (2000)
19. Nehmer, J., Becker, M., Karshmer, A., Lamm, R.: Living assistance systems: an ambient intelligence approach. In: Proceedings of the 28th International Conference on Software Engineering, pp. 43–50. ACM, New York (2006)
20. Perry, B.D.: Incubated in Terror: Neurodevelopmental Factors in the Cycle of Violence. In: Children, Youth and Violence: The Search for Solutions, pp. 124–148. Guilford Press, New York (1997)
21. Siegel, D.J.: The Developing Mind: How Relationships and the Brain Interact to Shape Who We are. The Guilford Press, New York (1999)
22. Spielberger, C.D.: State-Trait Anxiety Inventory for Children, STAIC, Palo Alto (1973)

Review and New Proposals for Zigbee Applications in Healthcare and Home Automation

Iker Caballero, Javier Vicente Sáez, and Begoña García Zapirain

DeustoTech-Life Unit, Deusto Institute of Technology,
University of Deusto,
Avda. de las Universidades, 24. 48007 Bilbao, Spain
{iker.caballero,jvicente,mbgarciazapi}@deusto.es

Abstract. The DeustoTech-Life research group at University of Deusto is developping a health monitoring system. This system is intended to make life easier not only for the elderly but also for people with chronic diseases, providing a way of keeping daily records of biomedical measurements The main aim of this work is to promote the standardization and interoperability of this kind of applications, because recent projects do not meet the standard perfectly. The proposal is to develop the ZigBee Cluster Library to achieve this aim so that the devices can be interoperable and standards. The results will be the development of a fully interoperable health monitoring system and the design of new ZCL compliant health devices.

Keywords: ZigBee, healthcare, interoperability, standardization.

1 Introduction

Many projects on domotics have been carried out in recent years, but the technologies used to design these systems have either been updated or have depreciated. The fact is that new technologies have appeared to offer opportunities in developing new and better applications in this area [1].

Several of these projects have focused on the elderly and independent life [2][3], but there are no such solutions for healthcare, which involves not only the elderly but also people with chronic diseases or poor health [4].

All of them need to keep continuous records on any biometric parameter and then give them to the doctor to be studied or analyzed. Apart from an improvement in the quality of life they require, it is important to mention that most of these people cannot afford the life they need. The systems developed should be as cheap and complete as possible so that people can obtain them without problems of any kind. This goal can only be only achieved by developing standard-based systems such as the one propose in this paper.

Therefore, the technological solution presented in this paper intends to increase possibilities in terms of quality and independent life, leading to this collective of people not needing to be aware of the records all the time. The solution consists of a network divided into different parts according to their offered services: on the one hand, a standard domotic profile which involves switches, lights, dimmers, etc; and

J. Bravo, R. Hervás, and V. Villarreal (Eds.): IWAAL 2011, LNCS 6693, pp. 101–108, 2011.
© Springer-Verlag Berlin Heidelberg 2011

on the other hand, a healthcare profile in charge of controlling and monitoring health and biometric devices.

The main aim of this work is to promote the standardization and interoperability of this kind of application. This would increase the number of devices available and thus competition, leading to a reduction in price. In accordance with this aim, several specific aims can be highlighted:

— A standard-based system to reduce costs and permit interoperation between different manufacturers.

— Use of only one technology for domotics and healthcare.

— Developing an intuitive system offering a wide range of services focused on health and welfare.

— Design of new health devices with minimal user intervention to get them started.

2   Review of Wireless Sensor Networks in Social Applications

Wireless technologies have substantial advantages over wired ones. First of all, mobility is one of the most important advantages because it allows the user to be connected to the network over a wide area, not forgetting the technological limits as far as distance is concerned. In the case of a house, it is possible to develop a system that allows the user to connect to the network from any room.

Another advantage is the initial cost or the system installation costs, which are much lower compared to a wired network as it requires no work on the house, such as building work or painting. This is a significant saving since elderly often live in old houses that have no pre-installation of home automation wiring, as currently established by common telecommunication infrastructure standards. And finally, the scalability makes it possible to add new devices to the network without problems (always bearing in mind the limits of the technology used in terms of number of nodes).

We have to consider also the main disadvantages of wireless technologies such as power management. It is a pain to change batteries every week or month, so there are a lot of research about power-consumption and energy harvesting. Another point to keep in mind is the failure probability which increase proportionally to the number of devices in network.

2.1   Comparison of Wireless Technologies

Bluetooth has been the most widely-used wireless technology in domotics over the years [5] but, with the emergence of low-power technologies, it has been replaced by applications that require greater bandwidth and data rates,

ZigBee and ANT are two low-power consumption technologies that are in direct competition with each other. Although they have similar features regarding power and network capabilities, there are several differences that are the key to selecting one of them. Both of these technologies share the low-power consumption feature, unlike Bluetooth, but ANT has a significant feature –not a problem- that could be the reason for not choosing it: the standard on which it is based is proprietary. Although this feature might not be a problem developing a specific application, it is in terms of interoperating between manufacturers. You cannot add new devices to the network of other manufacturers unless this new manufacturer is based on the ANT proprietary standard, probably having to pay an expensive license. These and other differences between these three technologies are shown in Table 1.

Table 1. Wireless technologies comparison

Feature	ANT	ZigBee	Bluetooth
Standard	Proprietary	IEEE802.15.4	IEEE802.15.1
Application	PANs and WSNs	PANs and WSNs	PANs
Battery life	Years	Months/years	Days
Max. nodes	2^{32}	2^{64}	7
Tx rate (kbit/s)	1000	250	1000
Range	1 to 30m	>100m	1 to 10m
Topologies	P2P, star, tree, mesh	P2P, star, tree, mesh	P2P, star

2.2 ZigBee in Home Automation and Healthcare Applications

The technology selected for this project is ZigBee, which provides best performance and is based on IEEE802.15.4 standard, an exceptional advantage over ANT. ZigBee adds network and routing services to 802.15.4. It was developed in 2004, but its stack became obsolete as the 2006 and 2007 stack releases (also called ZigBee Pro) offer more network features but are not backward compatible [8]. These latter releases are not fully compatible between each other because routers of one release must act as end devices in the other, but they can work together without problems.

Furthermore, the ZigBee Alliance is a non-profit association whose main aim is to develop standards suiting the real evolving needs of manufacturers and developers. This is the reason why they work with companies that are members of the Alliance, certifying their devices as ZigBee certified products.

The Alliance designed some application profiles with industry experts to meet the market needs. They developed some profiles such as Home Automation [9] and Healthcare Profiles, both used in the suggested design. These profiles should help the developers to design interoperable devices by using the ZigBee Cluster Library (ZCL). This library provides the developer with a number of specific clusters (seen as functionalities) for each network device.

Specifically, the Home Automation Profile offers a global standard for smart homes, enabling them to control lighting, environment or security for instance. Smarter homes allow clients to save money and enjoy a variety of conveniences to improve quality and independent life. On the other hand, Health Care Profile has been designed to enable reliable monitoring of non-critical healthcare services, targeted as independent life, health and wellness, or chronic diseases. The smart devices designed under this profile could provide connection with doctors or nurses so that they may monitor the health of a patient even when at home. [10]

Apart from ZigBee Alliance, there is another non-profit organization called Continua Health Alliance, which boasts collaboration with the best companies in terms of electronics and health and medical devices (Intel, IBM, Nokia; Omron, Roche, etc). Their main aim is to establish a system of interoperable health solutions empowering individuals and providing personalized health and wellness management. [11]

The first release performed by Continua adopted Bluetooth as the communication standard technology for health devices. As ZigBee Alliance does, Continua Alliance certifies health devices under the Continua Health Guidelines. These Guidelines contain references to all standards and specs that Continua selected for ensuring interoperability [12].

2.3 Standardization Problems and Conclusions

These alliances that pursue the single goal of interoperability also encourage competitiveness between manufacturers, thus providing benefits for the market. Although keeping to the standard is the only way to enter the market, it is not as easy as we may think. Companies have to analyze their profitability and standardization is not the easiest and the cheapest way. But this is only the point of view from companies' domain.

Although a few years ago it was different, nowadays the focus is the end user, thus the costumer. The main target of companies should meet the needs of customers, and they are demanding systems that can integrate new features without having to buy new equipment and filling the house with lots of tech-gadgets. The standardization is the only way to achieve it.

3 New Proposals for an Ideal Scenario in Health Monitoring

As mentioned above, the ZigBee and ZigBee Pro versions are not compatible. Manufacturers place their ZigBee Certified logo on their products but we have to refer to the detailed specification to check if the product is ZigBee or ZigBee Pro certified. And if it is ZigBee Pro certified, it would not implement the complete cluster library (ZCL).

This is a major problem in development kits because application developers have to manage along the specification of the cluster library to implement it, thus delaying product design. Although ZCL is a clear specification, it is difficult to manage. You can easily become confused by the different profiles, clusters and their attributes. The addition of this new layer gives the ZigBee stack more complexity even though is a great aid to interoperability.

The continuous and fast advances in technology do not allow manufacturers to recover their investment in product designs, so these advances are delaying interoperability. New technologies have to appear absolutely specified, and the advances should be in horizontal form. If a specification satisfies all needs, it should be kept for a long time to allow manufacturers to recover their investment. This means, for example, that the standard specification should be clearly specified and closed in the ZigBee Alliance and they should only develop complementary clusters or profiles. If new complementary functionalities appear, the manufacturers could design new devices to expand their offer without wasting previous ones. And this is the way towards standardization; in other words, the way to interoperability. Besides, there are many designs that use gateways as a means of providing interoperability between different systems, but the ideal scenario should be developed with systems based on a single technology.

The main aim of this project is to implement a standard system which will be interoperable. For this purpose, the development of the ZCL layer is needed because most manufacturers have not developed it. If every manufacturer does the same, prices will fall. The current situation can be described in Fig. 1. There are three devices produced by different manufacturers, yet providing the same functionality. The prices are still high for a middle-class person and the cheapest one implements a proprietary layer over ZigBee Network Layer.

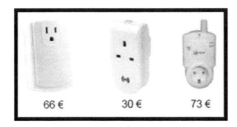

Fig. 1. ZigBee home plugs

Therefore, the first challenge is to achieve a standard system and to promote standardization so as to reduce costs. These costs should not be very important for the personal economy, but the social budget should cover them as most of these systems are installed via the Ministry or the Social Security.

Apart from the ZCL layer, a gateway interface must be developed between the network coordinator and the central monitoring station. This gateway will accept not only our devices but also devices from different manufacturers which are ZigBee Pro certified and ZCL compatible. The new devices that are being designed, will also work in other manufacturers' network systems.

The research group has chosen ZigBee as the wireless communication protocol. Therefore, all advantages will be taken from it, such as Smart Energy Profile to measure energy efficiency in home plugs or the RSSI and LQI values for indoor localization. Although there is no connection between these features and the Healthcare Profile, it is important to take advantage of all the services offered by the technology.

Another part of the project is the design of new devices in both Home Automation and Healthcare Profiles. In terms of home automation, we are designing switches and appliance modules, light dimmers, etc. Although there are a lot of these products on the market, they are not fully ZigBee compatible, and we intend to add the Smart Energy Profile to them in order to provide data on energy consumption.

In terms of healthcare, we are trying to analyze which devices could be designed starting from scratch and which ones can be adapted to ZigBee technology. In the first case, new sensors will be implemented. And, it is not advisable to spend time on the latter case if reliable devices have already been designed. We will add ZigBee wireless transmission to them so that they can be incorporated into our system. The next release of Continua Design Guidelines is planned to be over ZigBee Standard due to its benefits versus Bluetooth (low-power consumption, mesh topology support, etc.) so, another big challenge for this project is that of getting everything ready when this happens. As well as the general opportunities in consumer and health electronics, it is important to predict the direction taken by these systems to anticipate future needs.

We have to mention that these devices should be prototypes in order to test the system features and if they meet the needs of end users. As a research department of a company does, our aim is to study if these approaches meet the needs. The aim is not to bring these devices to market, so a lot o rules and regulations will be bypassed. We have just to take them into account when the product will be sold.

In conclusion, the standardization will enable interoperation between our system and other manufacturers' products if they are ZigBee certified. The system will promote self care, independent living, as well as wellness and fitness. It will also provide a base system where new profiles and services could be added, such as panic buttons or fall detectors on a healthcare plane but focused on security.

4 Results

Although this is work in progress, we have obtained satisfactory results in what has been done. The software line has focused on completing the ZigBee Pro Stack of the acquired development kit, more specifically, developing the ZCL layer of the protocol. This layer is needed to design new devices that meet ZigBee profiles, including Home Automation or Healthcare ones. The layer grows according to the needs (the horizontal growth mentioned above).

Besides, a transparent serial protocol has been developed, one which enables any embedded device to communicate with the network controller, thus allowing management of the ZigBee network. This protocol has been designed with an AT-like structure.

In the hardware part, several devices have been designed to meet the HA profile, such as:

- Switch.
- On/Off module.
- Dimmer.
- Panic button.

We have tested the end devices with our coordinator and others to verify that they are interoperable. In addition, network traffic captures have sniffed to verify they meet the standard and to dismiss a lot of modules that have been acquired and are not ZCL compatible. Our coordinator has communicated with devices from other manufacturers, and our modules with other coordinators. We used a light-switch demo to verify if the controller and the devices were interoperable with the controller and between them. It would have been desirable to test devices from more manufacturers but, unfortunately, they are not fully standard compliant.

Besides the home automation devices, we have designed two prototypes of health devices: a galvanic resistance stress meter and an ECG monitor. These devices have been integrated into the sensor network using private profiles. Once the Healthcare Profile is completed, we will change them to this profile to achieve the main objective of having ZigBee compliant devices that can interoperate with other platforms, reaching a prototype as show in Fig. 2.

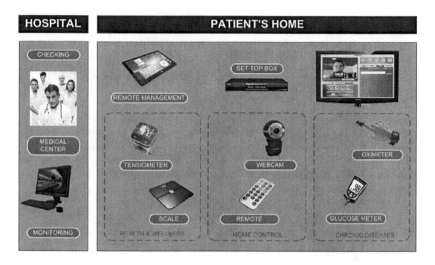

Fig. 2. Future system prototype

5 Conclusions

As has been argued throughout the paper, the DeustoTech-Life research group is working on the socialization of new technologies focused on healthcare and ambient-assisted living, taking standardization as the first step to achieve this socialization. In this case, the group pledged its commitment to using the profiles developed by the ZigBee Alliance. The group has designed devices that are ZigBee HA compliant and have been tested to verify their interoperability. As far as healthcare is concerned, two new devices have been designed but using private profiles. Once the Healthcare profile is complete, they will be migrated into it. We sincerely hope that our contribution will promote the adoption of standards as a way of socializing these technologies so useful for such important collectives of society: the elderly, people with special needs and those who have chronic diseases.

Considering future lines of work, the group has begun developing new sensors that measure specific parameters of several health problems, such as stress, breast cancer, and kidney problems among others. The fact of developing these sensors according to the standard mentioned in the paper allows their direct integration into any tele-medical system and therefore swift incorporation into any real pilot project with patients.

References

[1] Simons, D.P.L.: Consumer Electronics Opportunities in Remote and Home Healthcare. In: International Conference on Consumer Electronics, ICCE 2008, Digest of Technical Papers (2008)

[2] García, B., Ruiz, I., Vicente, J., Méndez, A.: BIOHOME: A House Designed for Assisted Living. In: IWAAL (2009)

[3] Vicente, J., García, B., Méndez, A., Eguiluz, G.: Biohome: Residential Gateway for People with Special Needs Remotely Controlled by Android Smartphone. In: IWAAL (2010)

[4] Casas, R., Marco, A., Plaza, I., Garrido, Y., Falco, J.: ZigBee-based alarm system for pervasive healthcare in rural. IET Communications 2, 208

[5] Zhang, Y., Xiao, H.: Bluetooth-Based Sensor Networks for Remotely Monitoring the Physiological Signals of a Patient. IEEE Transactions on Information Technology in Biomedicine 13, 1040–1048

[6] Lee, J.-S., Su, Y.-W., Shen, C.-C.: A Comparative Study of Wireless Protocols: Bluetooth, UWB, ZigBee, and Wi-Fi. In: 33rd Annual Conference of the IEEE. Industrial Electronics Society, IECON 2007 (2007)

[7] Evans-Pughe, C.: *Bzzzz zzz*[ZigBee wireless standard. IEE Review 49, 28–31

[8] Ling, P.: Mixed signals - ZigBee aims to be a standard for industrial low-power radio, but we might never see full compatibility between modules that support it. IET Electronics Systems and Software 5, 34–37

[9] Egan, D.: The emergence of ZigBee in building automation and industrial control. Computing & Control Engineering Journal 16, 14–19

[10] Sangani, K.: Home Automation – It's no place like home. Engineering & Technology 1, 46

[11] Wartena, F., Muskens, J., Schmitt, L.: Continua: The Impact of a Personal Telehealth Ecosystem. In: International Conference on eHealth, Telemedicine, and Social Medicine, eTELEMED 2009 (2009)

[12] Carroll, R., Cnossen, R., Schnell, M., Simons, D.: Continua: An Interoperable Personal Healthcare Ecosystem. IEEE Pervasive Computing 6, 90–94

AVATAR: An Open Source Architecture for Embodied Conversational Agents in Smart Environments

Marcos Santos-Pérez, Eva González-Parada, and José Manuel Cano-García

Electronic Technology Department, School of Telecommunications Engineering,
University of Malaga, Teatinos Campus, 29071 Malaga, Spain
{marcos_sape,gonzalez,jcgarcia}@uma.es

Abstract. Due to a growing older population, researchers and industry are paying more attention to the needs of this group of people. Ambient Intelligence (AmI) aims to help people in their daily lives, achieving a more natural interaction of users with an electronic home environment. Embodied Conversational Agents (ECAs) arise as a natural interface between humans and AmI. Our contribution is to present AVATAR: an architecture to develop ECAs based on open source tools and libraries. In the current prototype the virtual agent acts as a natural control interface of the home automation system. In addition, we provide the details to allow its use by Spanish speakers.

1 Introduction

World population ageing is caused by lower overall mortality and fertility. The older population is growing at an enormous pace. In absolute terms the number of older persons has tripled since 1950 and is expected to triple again by 2050 [8].

Older people want to maintain as much independence as possible in their lives. Ambient Assisted Living (AAL) aims to make life easier for people in their own homes by using a set of advanced electronic sensors and automated devices.

A major trend in the development of interfaces for intelligent environments is the use of Embodied Conversational Agents (ECAs) who act as mediators [5]. The daily use of such interfaces creates an illusion of collaboration and may develop social and emotional ties to these virtual assistants. Another interesting application for ECAs is the management of the user's medical needs in their own homes[15]. Research has found that face to face conversation with an embodied agent increases the participation with the system [17]. Furthermore, the presentation of content through the use of a virtual agent improves the ability to retain information [2].

Different architectures for ECAs have been proposed through the integration of various programs and corporate tools [19] [1]. This article focuses on the description of an open source and free architecture for ECAs named AVATAR. The vast majority of research in the eld of ECAs assume the use of English between the user and the system but our prototype works in Spanish due to its worldwide distribution.

This paper is organized as follows: after this introduction, Section 2 describes the architecture of our AVATAR platform. The most important aspects of each component of the platform are explained in each subsection. Section 3 summarizes the conclusions drawn from the paper and discusses the future improvements of AVATAR.

J. Bravo, R. Hervás, and V. Villarreal (Eds.): IWAAL 2011, LNCS 6693, pp. 109–115, 2011.

2   AVATAR Platform Architecture

In this section we describe the actual implementation of the AVATAR platform. Figure 1 shows its block diagram. It consists of the following basic components:

- *Voice Activity Detector (VAD)* discriminates voice against environmental noise.
- *Automatic Speech Recognition (ASR)* performs speech to text conversion.
- *Conversational Engine (CE)* extracts the meaning, controls the dialog flow and produces a semantic representation suitable for the task context. It generates a response based on the input, the current state of conversation and dialog history.
- *Task Manager (TM)* connects to the environmental devices.
- *Text-To-Speech (TTS)* generates the output speech signal and the timing configuration for the virtual head animation.
- *Virtual Head Animation (VHA)* sets the facial animation synchronized with the output speech.

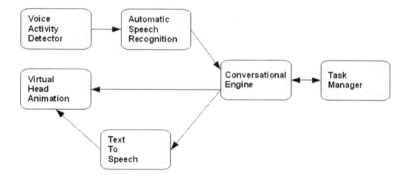

Fig. 1. AVATAR architecture

The architecture follows a modular design so that each component of the platform can be modified without affecting others. Each component runs in a different thread and communicates with the next by a message queue.

2.1   Voice Activity Detector

The VAD role is to differentiate the audio segments where the user speaks from those containing noise. VAD are usually used in other scenarios, such as mobile communications and Voice over IP (VoIP). In these scenarios, the VAD function aims to achieve a reduction of network traffic in order to save bandwith. Although the operating principles are the same, the purpose of the VAD in conversational interfaces is to segment the user's speech into sentences.

The VAD is fed directly with the digitized samples coming from the microphone and sends the raw audio from the segments containing user's voice to the ASR.

The most common VAD algorithms are based on energy threshold and zero crossing rate of the signal. In our platform this role is performed by the SphinxBase library [7].

2.2   Automatic Speech Recognition

Voice recognition is a crucial part of the conversational system and its functionality is essential to allow voice communication between human beings and electronic systems.

The complexity of such systems lies in the diversity of factors that includes human speech (acoustics, phonetics, phonology, lexicon, semantics). In many cases, the sense of naturalness of the conversational interface depends heavily on the robustness of speech recognition [14]. Despite these difficulties some notable advances in this field have been achieved in recent years and make possible automatic speech recognition with acceptable error levels for a large number of applications [23].

The recognizer can be viewed as a black box that transforms the voice segments that come from the VAD directly to text, which is sent to the CE.

In our AVATAR platform, speech recognition is performed by PocketSphinx library, which belongs to the CMU Sphinx family [6]. The reasons for this choice are that this library allows speaker-independent speech recognition and has been used in real-time applications [12].

Voice recognition needs both an acoustic and a language corpus to run. For this project, we used the Voxforge Spanish corpus [21]. It is the first free speaker-independent acoustic model for spanish. The statistical language model in the prototype is generated from a set of possible sentences that led to a dictionary of 75 different words to control the various elements of the simulated environment.

2.3   Conversational Engine

Classic conversational agents usually lead to too linear and rigid talks. For a more natural feel and in order to avoid being rejected by users, it is necessary that the system can handle unexpected changes of context and be able to achieve many goals asynchronously [13]. One approach to this type of systems with great success in both academic and commercial sector is that of conversational bots.

A chatbot or conversational bot is a program that simulates a conversation with someone. There are currently a large number of chatterbots or chatbots used in various fields [16] such as marketing, education [4] or entertainment. One of the most remarkable is "ELIZA" [22], which is considered the forerunner of the current conversational bots. The most successful chatbots seem to be based on AIML, an XML-based language that is considered a de facto standard after its composition and operation were published.

The conversational engine of AVATAR platform is based on PyAIML [20]. It is an open source AIML interpreter and it is fully compatible with AIML 1.0.1 standard.

The CE module receives the text from the ASR and draws its possible meaning. In our prototype its main objective is to obtain the values that fill the slots needed for the TM. These slots correspond to the action to take, the type of object that receives the action, the name of the object, the change of the object state and the room where the object is. In addition, the CE module must also manage the context and history of the conversation since the user is free to provide all necessary data at one time or not. With this information the CE module communicates with the TM and generates a textual response understandable to the user informing him the result of his action or requesting for further information.

2.4   Task Manager

The task manager provides an interface between the conversational engine and the smart home.

While the ECA can run on a handheld device, the control system of the house is usually implemented in a desktop computer. Therefore, the task manager provides a client-server architecture. The client module runs on the same machine as the ECA and then sends requests to the home. On the other hand, the server module translates the requests into the language of the home automation system and responds with confirmation or error messages or to the agent.

In the current development stage of the AVATAR project automation control system is simulated. Figure 2 graphically displays the status of various objects that can be managed on the server.

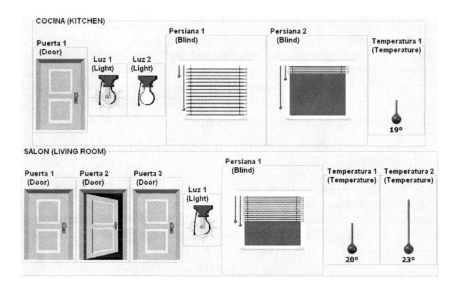

Fig. 2. Simulated devices controlled on the server

2.5   Text-To-Speech

There are different methods for obtaining a synthetic voice and each has advantages and disadvantages. Concatenative synthesis is achieved by attaching pre-recorded voice segments. For specific application domain it is often preferred to store whole words, which leads to a high quality artificial voice. Instead formant synthesis produces the sound wave varying physical parameters of an acoustic model. By not using human voice segments, it produces a robotic voice and its usage only makes sense in systems with limited hardware resources. There are other types of synthesis, but they are not yet matured enough for its use in complete systems.

The TTS module just needs the response text from the CE to synthesize the artificial voice. Just before starting the playback of the response it sends the data with the duration of each vocal segment to the VHA module.

The TTS system used in AVATAR is Festival [10]. Festival TTS is an open source synthesizer of free use from the University of Edinburgh. Festival offers a robust synthesis algorithm based on concatenation of diphonemes. It currently supports both English and Spanish.

The default voice in Spanish of Festival does not offer a high quality, so we opted to use the male voice from the Hispavoces project of the Andalusian Regional Government [11].

2.6 Virtual Head Animation

The virtual head is the embodiment of intelligent agent. A usual rule of avatar design states that the realism of its appearance must correspond with its behavior. Otherwise, the avatar will be rejected because of what is known as the Uncanny Valley effect [9]. For this reason an effort was made to give it the greatest possible realism. The head model includes 22 different bones and has more than 30 different animated expressions in addition to the 10 visemes that are needed to simulate speech.

The response text from CE and the duration of the audio segments from the TTS module are the needed entries for the animation of the virtual head. The technique used to achieve lip synchronization is as follows. The first step is to conduct a preliminary analysis of the response text generated by the conversational engine in order to obtain the list of visemes to be executed simultaneously with the audio. The second step is to modulate the playback speed of each visema animation depending on the length of each segment of the sentence. It is worth noting that the selection of facial expressions during the speech animation is still under development.

Head modeling and animation were made with Blender [3]. Blender is a multi-platform software application that specializes in 3D graphics modeling and animation. Released as free software under the GNU General Public License, Blender is available for a number of operating systems, including GNU/Linux, Mac OS X, FreeBSD, OpenBSD and Microsoft Windows.

OGRE [18] is used as rendering engine in AVATAR. It is a scene-oriented 3D rendering engine written in C++. The class library abstracts the details of using the underlying system libraries like Direct3D and OpenGL and provides an interface based on world objects and other high-level classes. Released under the terms of the MIT License, the engine is free software.

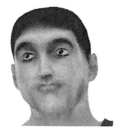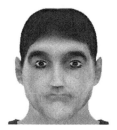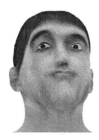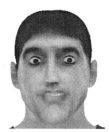

Fig. 3. Virtual head in different poses

3   Conclusion and Future Work

The main goal of this work was to describe a software platform aimed at developing ECAs. Thus, we proposed a possible design and defined the architecture and implementation details for such platform. We made an extra effort during the election of the components to be integrated so we could obtain a free and open source platform.

Currently, the platform is still under development, so hopefully the final version will present improvements over the version described in this document.

A line of future work focuses on modeling users through Case-Based Reasoning (CBR). In order to automatically identify the speaker it can be used a classic technique of pattern matching based on the features of the user's voice.

A second line of future work is related to the integration of the whole platform in an embedded system in order to use it in new user devices like mobile phones or tablet computers.

Acknowledgments

This work was partially supported with public funds by the Spanish National Project TEC2009-13763-C02-01 and by the Andalusian Regional Project P08-TIC4198.

References

1. Baldassarri, S., Cerezo, E., Serón, F.: An open source engine for embodied animated agents. In: XVII Congreso Español de Informática Gráfica (CEIG 2007), Zaragoza, Spain, pp. 91–98 (September 2007)
2. Beun, R.-J., de Vos, E., Witteman, C.: Embodied conversational agents: Effects on memory performance and anthropomorphisation. In: Rist, T., Aylett, R.S., Ballin, D., Rickel, J. (eds.) IVA 2003. LNCS (LNAI), vol. 2792, pp. 315–319. Springer, Heidelberg (2003)
3. Blender website, http://www.blender.org
4. Burguillo-Rial, J.C., Rodríguez-Silva, D.A., Santos-Pérez, M.: T-Bot: an intelligent tutoring agent for open e-Learning platforms. In: 8th International Conference on Information Technology Based Higher Education and Training (ITHET 2007), Kumamoto City, Japan (July 2007)
5. Carolis, B.D., Mazzotta, I., Novielli, N., Pizzutilo, S.: Social robots and ECAs for accessing smart environments services. In: Proceedings of the International Conference on Advanced Visual Interfaces, AVI 2010, pp. 275–278. ACM, New York (2010)
6. CMU Sphinx website, http://cmusphinx.sourceforge.net/
7. CMU Sphinxbase website, http://sourceforge.net/projects/cmusphinx/
8. D. of Economic and Social Affairs. Population Division. World population ageing 2009. Tech. rep., United Nations
9. Fabri, M.: Emotionally Expressive Avatars for Collaborative Virtual Environments. PhD thesis, Leeds Metropolitan University, Leeds, UK (November 2006)
10. Festival Speech Synthesis System website, http://www.cstr.ed.ac.uk/projects/festival/
11. Guadalinex Hispavoces website, http://forja.guadalinex.org/frs/?group_id=21

12. Huggins-daines, D., Kumar, M., Chan, A., Black, A.W., Ravishankar, M., Rudnicky, A.I.: PocketSphinx: a free, real-time continuous speech recognition system for hand-held devices. In: Proc. of ICASSP, Touluse, France, pp. 185–188 (May 2006)
13. Hung, V., Gonzalez, A., Demara, R.: Towards a Context-Based dialog management layer for expert systems. In: International Conference on Information, Process, and Knowledge Management, eKNOW 2009, Cancun, Mexico, pp. 60–65 (February 2009)
14. Jokinen, K.: Natural language and dialogue interfaces. In: The Universal Access Handbook, 1st edn., pp. 495–506. CRC Press Taylor & Francis Group (2009)
15. Kenny, P., Parsons, T., Gratch, J., Rizzo, A.: Virtual humans for assisted health care. In: Proceedings of the 1st international conference on PErvasive Technologies Related to Assistive Environments, PETRA 2008, pp. 6:1–6:4. ACM, New York (2008)
16. Kowalski, S., Pavlovska, K., Goldstein, M.: Two case studies in using chatbots for security training. Brazil (2009)
17. Mulken, S.V., André, E., Müller, J.: The persona effect: How substantial is it? In: Proceedings of HCI on People and Computers XIII, HCI 1998, pp. 53–66. Springer, London (1998)
18. OGRE website, http://www.ogre3d.org
19. Pejsa, T., Pandzic, I.S.: Architecture of an animation system for human characters. In: Proceedings of the 10th International Conference on Telecommunications, ConTEL 2009, pp. 171–176. IEEE, Zagreb (2009)
20. PyAIML. A Python AIML Interpreter website, http://pyaiml.sourceforge.net/
21. Voxforge Spanish Model website,
    http://cmusphinx.sourceforge.net/2010/08/
    voxforge-spanish-model-released/
22. Weizenbaum, J.: ELIZA: computer program for the study of natural language communication between man and machine. Commun. ACM 9(1), 36–45 (1966)
23. Zhang, J., Ward, W., Pellom, B., Yu, X., Hacioglu, K.: Improvements in audio processing and language modeling in the CU communicator. In: Eurospeech 2001, Aalborg, Denmark (September 2001)

Cognitive Wireless Sensor Network Device for AAL Scenarios

Fernando López, Elena Romero, Javier Blesa,
Daniel Villanueva, and Alvaro Araujo

Electronic Engineering Department, Universidad Politécnica de Madrid
Avda/ Complutense 30,
28040 Madrid, Spain
{flopez,elena,jblesa,danielvg,araujo}@die.upm.es

Abstract. Cognitive Networks appear as solution to avoid AAL scenarios problems like wireless interferences, secure a reliable communications, power consumption or different Quality of Service application needs. In this paper a prototype for Cognitive Wireless Sensor Networks is presented. This node is a hardware solution that will help to overcome problems in AAL Sensors Networks. The prototype, with three different radio interfaces, is looking for creating a network which can auto-optimize communications in real time related to different application needs. This solution allows developers to implement new applications and services for AAL scenarios.

Keywords: Cognitive Network, wireless interface, WSN, collaboration.

1 Motivation

AALIANCE [1] has defined an Ambient Assisted Living roadmap based on architectures with services obtained for the aggregation of Wireless Personal Area Networks (WPAN), Local Area Networks (LAN) and Wireless Area Networks (WAN) interfaces. AALIANCE encourages building inter-operable systems that can work together. To carry this out, interoperability in the following areas is needed: physical, connectivity, protocols, and services. AAL developers have to pay attention to hardware, communications and radio challenges.

In most cases AAL scenarios have been developed using wireless network architectures. Usually, these scenarios use Wireless Sensor Networks (WSN) solutions which operate in ISM unlicensed spectrum bands.

Unlicensed radio spectrum is becoming overcrowded. WSN have problems related to Quality of Service (QoS), efficiency and power consumption as a result of a huge number of devices using wireless communications like WiFi, Bluetooth, ZigBee...

Cognitive Radio (CR) is a software and hardware solution which can help to solve AAL scenario problems. With this solution a network or a wireless node can change their transmission or reception parameters. CR solutions are based on the active monitoring of external and internal radio environment including radio frequency spectrum, user behavior and network state. CR communicates efficiently avoiding interference with different users.CR solutions are focused on lower protocol layers in

J. Bravo, R. Hervás, and V. Villarreal (Eds.): IWAAL 2011, LNCS 6693, pp. 116–121, 2011.

spite of CN solution which is focused in high level protocol layers. Mitola introduced this idea in 1999 [2].

Cognitive Networks (CN) appears as the paradigm to avoid these problems. CN are based on three technical issues: cognitive capabilities of nodes, collaboration among terminals and learn about your history. This network is seen as a communication network that can span vertically over layers (making use of cross-layer design) and horizontally across nodes (covering a heterogeneous environment). It has to take decisions and need at least two elements:

- A representation of relevant knowledge about the network status like channels noise, CPU status of each node, operative sensors...
- A cognition loop which uses Artificial Intelligence (AI) techniques (learning and decision making techniques, etc.).

We propose to extend the CN paradigm to WSN to use more efficiently communication channels, reduce power consumption, and increase security and reliability. These features are very useful to overcome communication problems in AAL scenarios.

Our first approach has been to design a Cognitive Wireless Sensor Network node prototype. The goal is to test and find new optimization algorithms depending of different constraints (power optimization, QoS, cost, reliability...).

The prototype is a real solution made of commercial technologies. It is able to create a very flexible CN which can be used to solve different scenarios because of their different radio interfaces and capabilities of sharing and processing data.

In this paper we propose a CN hardware solution to approach to the design of AAL applications. In Section 2 we review some of the most relevant approaches. In Section 3 the node prototype will be described. In section 4 an AAL scenario to use the technology is presented. Finally, in Section 5, some conclusions and future work will be shown.

2 Related Work

There are no many technical works which combine AAL and CN. In [3] authors compare WSN simulations introducing two scenarios. In the first scenario they use a CR and Dynamic Spectrum Access (DSA) model. In the second one, they use a ZigBee model. This paper is focused on problems like incumbent's detection and user QoS. The results show bigger ranges in CR solution because of capability of using lower frequencies than ZigBee. Author also notes that recovery procedures have to be studied.

A theoretical study in [4] speaks about Cognitive Wireless Sensors Networks (CWSN). Challenges like energy efficiency and delay are introduced. They are caused by sensing time and how to use it to handle different data sources.

In [5] the existing communication protocols and algorithms devised for cognitive radio networks and WSNs are discussed along with the open research avenues for the realization of Cognitive Radio Sensors Networks (CRSN).

In [6] a CR-WSN solution is discussed like a next-generation WSN. The authors focus on designing challenges of CR-WSNs. The paper provides an overview and conceptual design of WSNs from the perspective of CR. It emphasizes the importance of creating a prototype that works as a deployment platform.

We have been looking for a node that applies CN paradigm to WSN and there is no possible to find a commercial or work in progress about this. Our node is a new way to investigate a real hardware solution in WSN solutions for AAL scenarios.

3 Node Description

There are a lot of different wireless network solutions to solve each specific problem. Therefore in AAL scenario too many different wireless solutions fight inefficiently for using a spectrum region. In order to find a global solution a prototype of CN node has been built.

The test platform is looking for optimizing communications in real time related to different application needs. So the CN has to consider power consumption, data rate, reliability and security in order to be useful to AAL applications.

There are almost six main problems which is mandatory to solve:

- Interferences with other wireless devices or noise problems have to been avoid, which implies that nodes have to change their frequency and modulation as fast as possible. For this reason the prototype has three different networks interfaces. Each node is capable of using different channels, and different kind of modulations.
- Power consumption is a very important challenge. Nowadays mobile and wear devices are used in AAL scenarios. As a consequence the system uses a low consumption microcontroller and wireless protocol. All the devices can switch off radio interfaces and sleep the cpu.
- Different security strategies for guarantee strong data integrity are needed. So the nodes have to change frequency, route traffic and add high level encryption methods.
- Cognitive Networks need to connect to different kind of regular commercial devices or internet gateways.
- To handle different data rates that fit to several applications. So node handles various data rates.
- Finally, it is needed to guarantee the reliability if a node is down or some interface is broken. So the network has to route the traffic. According to this, CN nodes are able to share information and synchronize the communication interfaces.

A prototype of Cognitive Network node has been designed according to these features. This prototype has to be capable of collecting data about the state of the network and to share the information with other nodes. In addition, each node will be able to change protocol parameters, protocols and wireless interfaces in real time so it is mandatory to coordinate all the network devices.

The test platform has been build using a microcontroller and three different radio interfaces because it is necessary to face many different situations and it need a lot of flexibility.

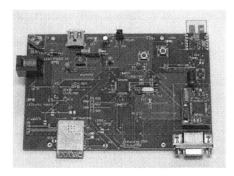

Fig. 1. Cognitive Wireless Sensor Network Device prototype

The control function is made by a Microchip PIC32MX795F512H, a 32-bit flash microcontroller. This is the higher performance processor which is low consumption and low cost. In addition Microchip provides a lot of protocol stacks, drivers and a good development environment.

CN node has three radio interfaces:

- A WiFi Microchip device which can handle data rate of 2Mbps and uses a band operation between 2.412 GHz - 2.484 GHz. WiFi is based on the IEEE 802.11 standards. In addition it is used by hundred devices so the Cognitive Networks can connect to client devices, external servers or LAN networks. This wireless chip can handle higher data rates than typical WSN.
- Other radio interface is MiWi protocol, designed by Microchip. It handles data rates about 250kbps and uses a band operation between 2.405-2.48 GHz. This is a proprietary wireless protocol that uses small, low-power digital radios based on the IEEE 802.15.4 standard for WPAN. It is designed for low data transmission rates and short distance, cost constrained networks.
- Last interface is uMercurio which is based on Texas Instruments CC1010 which can handle data rate of 76.8kbps and uses a band operation around 868 Mhz. uMercurio is a device developed by AWD (Universidad Politécnica de Madrid spin-off). It implements a communication protocol which works in a different band in contrast to the other interfaces. So it adds to our communication nodes bandwidth flexibility. Also this is a very low power solution.

Furthermore, the system also has RS-232 and USB communication interfaces. They are used like a computer interface to control the nodes.

Software has to recognize other nodes, sense the radio-electric environment, exchange configuration information, establish communication, and switch on or off the radio interfaces and sleep or wake up the nodes. The CN system is capable to prior emergency communication over other kind of traffic. In addition the use of batteries guarantees that the system works when there are electrical issues.

When this work in progress finish a flexible low consumption network with a distribution cognition processing will be working. This CN manages data routes optimizing consumption, data rate, reliability and security. As a result overcrowded unlicensed spectrum will be reduced. The system will be capable of connecting to internet throw WiFi, and using it like a gateway to make the CN global.

4 AAL Scenarios

A very interesting scenario related to use of CN in AAL environments is a big building which needs a lot of sensors working in a cooperative way: temperature, humidity, light. In addition there is a security system in the building which sends a picture each 5 seconds. There are also a lot of users in this building who has different needs, for example there are people who need a home monitoring system because of their blood pressure, pulse oximetry, ECG, etc. As example, we are going to show prototype contributions to this scenario.

A WSN solution can handle temperature, humidity and light sensors but it is not able to handle high data rates, so it can support a security system which use high quality pictures.

All these needs could be supported by a WiFi solution but it is impossible to guarantee low consumption when high data rates does not need.

Booth solutions cannot avoid strong noise problems because of using very close communication channels.

Our CN node is able to handle all applications. It can send high quality pictures or even IP voice because of WiFi interface. In addition the network can use low consumption radio interfaces if high bandwidth is not needed so we can increase batteries life more than other solutions. If It will be impossible to use the 2.4 Ghz unlicensed spectrum our device is able to use 868 Mhz band increasing reliability.

Medical data must be sent to a telemedicine server. With our CN node it is possible to connect an ECG sensor in a smart phone. The phone is link to a CN through WiFi and sends the information to a remote medical application. If a blackout happens it can guarantee connection and QoS because of the batteries. In addition the same network continues sensing and processing temperature, humidity and light sensors. As a result of blackout the CN could send a mail to the network administrator reporting about the situation. If some frequencies were overloaded, each node decide to change their channels or protocol agree to other nodes. In addition if some nodes were broken the network changes data routes and channels to guarantee a reliable communication. Finally, if the batteries level goes down idle nodes sleep as much time as possible and use the lowest power consumption network interface.

An efficient, low cost and reliable emergency security system can be implemented using the CN, therefore a lot different solutions can work together using the same low cost wireless network.

5 Conclusions and Future Work

Nowadays AAL scenarios solutions are implemented using many different WPAN solutions without interaction. Because of this lack of interoperability radio spectrum is inefficiently managed. A CN solution solves these problems because CN offers an intelligent network which can decide the best way to optimize all communications. Therefore there is essential to build a CN node prototype which use actual WPAN technology. This hardware has to sense the network, shares information and take decisions about how to manage communications. The goal is to build a cheap, low power, versatile CN node which can link to Internet, creating an auto configuration network and managing different kind of sensors or applications.

System is different to commercial solutions because it use three radio interfaces and it is able to synchronize each node. In addition it route or select radio interfaces following different rules.

We have built a new CN Wireless Sensor Network node with the above features to implement different optimization protocols. This node allows developers to implement new applications and services for AAL scenario as we present in Section 4.

In the future the platform will be improved. New functionality will be added and we include the prototype in a real scenario.

Acknowledgments. This work was funded by the Spanish Ministry of Industry, Tourism and Trade, under Research Grant TSI-020301-2009-18 (eCID), the Spanish Ministry of Science and Innovation, under Research Grant TEC2009-14595-C02-01, and the CENIT Project Segur@.

References

1. Van de Broek, G., Cavallo, F., Odetti, L., Wehrmann, C.: Ambient Assisted Living Roadmap: VDI/VDE-IT. In: AALIANCE Office, Berlin (2009)
2. Mitola III, J., Maguire Jr., G.Q.: Cognitive radio: making software radios more personal. IEEE Personal Communications, 13–18 (1999)
3. Cavalcanti, D., Das, S., Wang, J., Challapali, K.: Cognitive Radio Based Wireless Sensor Networks. In: Proceedings of 17th International Conference on Computer Communications and Networks, ICCCN 2008, pp. 1–6 (2008)
4. Zahmati, A.S., Hussain, S., Fernando, X., Grami, A.: Cognitive Wireless Sensor Networks: Emerging topics and recent challenges. In: 2009 IEEE Toronto International Conference of Science and Technology for Humanity (TIC-STH), pp. 593–596 (2009)
5. Akan, O., Karli, O., Ergul, O.: Cognitive radio sensor networks. IEEE Network 23(4), 34–40 (2009)
6. Yau, K.-L.A., Komisarczuk, P., Teal, P.D.: Cognitive Radio-based Wireless Sensor Networks: Conceptual design and open issues. In: Local Computer Networks, LCN 2009, pp. 955–962 (2009)

An Ambient Assisted Living Platform to Integrate Biometric Sensors to Detect Respiratory Failures for Patients with Serious Breathing Problems

Antonio J. Jara, Miguel A. Zamora, and Antonio F. Gómez Skarmeta

Computer Science Faculty, University of Murcia, Murcia, Spain
{jara,mzamora,skarmeta}@um.es

Abstract. Breathing problems such as chronic obstructive pulmonary disease, chronic bronchitis or emphysema, present the need to carry out home respiratory therapy. This requires the deployment of specific devices for supplemental oxygen therapy and monitoring of the status of the patient. This paper presents an Ambient Assisted Living solution to carry out the treatments in their houses. This introduces technological innovations and advanced services to allow patient monitoring and supervision by remote monitoring centers. This paper shows the developed architecture, where the selected biomedical sensors for monitoring the reduction in breathing capacity have been integrated. The platform permits to connect wirelessly the sensors worn by the patient to the gateway deployed at the house, and the safe and global communication and secure communication with the remote monitoring centers and Intelligent Information Systems. This improves the current solutions presented, where only 42% of the patients, who receive this therapy satisfy at least 80% of the therapy prescribed by the pulmonologist. Since, this solution supervises continuously the compliance of the patient to the respiratory therapy.

Keywords: COPD, home respiratory therapy, e-Health, Internet of Things, 6LoWPAN, Ambient Assisted Living.

1 Introduction

The remote monitoring is a requirement to support the new generation of healthcare solutions based on Ambient Assisted Living environments (AAL). In particular, this work presents an AAL solution for the detection of respiratory failures in patients with serious breathing problems, where it is more evident the need to carry out assistance and the therapy in the patient's house or specialized centers.

The solution presented is being defined in the frame of the Spanish project AIRE, whose goal is to design and develop a platform to support remote monitoring, and an intelligent system to detect and predict anomalies in the patients with serious breathing problems. Specifically, the goal of the system is to detect when the breathing capacity is being reduced, in order to warn to the caregivers to avoid insufficient respiratory, which can cause serious health problems and situations each time more dangerous, resulting even in some occasions in an irreversible consequence.

J. Bravo, R. Hervás, and V. Villarreal (Eds.): IWAAL 2011, LNCS 6693, pp. 122–130, 2011.
© Springer-Verlag Berlin Heidelberg 2011

Nowadays, in the market can be found some projects and solutions to support home respiratory therapy, but they are partial solutions, where for example it is only supported the home oxygen therapy or the remote monitoring of some biometric sensors, where the collected data need to be interpreted by the specialist or caregiver. Other solutions are focused on a specific illness, instead of offer a generic framework with support of sensors for monitoring parameters from very different kind of sensors. For example, it can be found specific solution to measure the lung capacity with a spirometer, and more advance solutions are focused on pilot deployments, which are not yet arrived to a commercial solution [1]. Specifically, the most relevant related solutions found are, on the one hand, the project Medic4all [2] for monitoring of patients with chronic obstructive pulmonary disease (COPD) in Israel, with a pilot deployment of 1200 patients. This solution transfers the monitored data wireless in real time to two remote monitoring centers. This considers a basic alarm system based on the status of the parameters, this alarm system warns to the caregivers/specialists when an anomalous value is found, in order to visit to the patient. This project is only focused on the first level of COPD solutions, i.e. monitoring level. On the other hand, the solution Health Buddy System [3], presents a system for monitoring of multiple diseases, where is also considered COPD. The experiments with this system, in a living lab of 59 patients, have demonstrated that the patients monitored with this kind of solutions have presented a lower quantity of side effects, health problems and the ratio of hospitalizations has been reduced [4]. Both projects are not considering a second level of solutions focused on intelligent systems with predict models to detect anomalies before that present serious symptoms and health problems such as the mentioned insufficient respiratory. Our approach is focused on the definition of an intelligent system to predict the mentioned situations with continuous analysis of the collected information from the health status and the context (e.g. activity of the patient).

Therefore, the goal in this project is to reach an intelligent system to link some respiratory parameters such as oxygen saturation (SpO2) levels, breathing frequency, lung capacity and peak expiratory flow (PEF) with the anomalies, as such to detect breathing problems previously to reach a bad situation. Thereby, the risk of problem is reduced as is the suffering from the patient in these situations.

This solution is based on the technologies from the Internet of Things to make possible the connection of the sensors worn by the patient in their environment with the Intelligent Information System (IIS) and monitoring centers through Internet.

The IIS is currently a work in progress, which has been designed to detect the patterns and models of the different respiratory illness, in function of the collected data from the biometric sensors and context information from the platform.

This paper is focused on present the defined architecture based on the Internet of Things, which has been designed to support the continuous monitoring of the patient for the collection of the data, which will be required by the IIS, as such as the integration of the biometric sensors in the architecture, with the final purpose of be able to offer the respiratory assistance services required to supply adequate oxygen therapy in AAL environments.

2   Home Respiratory Therapy

World Health Organization (WHO) statistics determine that 210 million people around the world suffer chronic obstructive pulmonary disease (COPD), over 3 million deaths, i.e. 5% of the deaths around the world were caused by COPD in 2005 [5]. In Spain, more than 4 million people suffer COPD, who are 9% of the population, following the statistics from the Spanish Society of neumonology and thorax cirugy, and over 18,000 of these people die per year in Spain, following the National Spanish Institute of Statistics. Remark, that from the mentioned patients in Spain, 80% of them have not been diagnosticated, since they consider the symptoms as "normal" because of tobacco consumption. The main reason for these problems in Spain is because 26.4% of the population consumes tobacco regularly, which triggers an abnormal inflammatory response in the lung.

Right now, there are more than 300,000 patients, who are receiving respiratory therapy at their homes in Spain. The increase in the appearance of the breathing illness and the aging of the population are some of the factors which show the need for the next years of the Ambient Assisted Living (AAL) as the solution to satisfy the demand and requirements of the healthcare in the near future.

In particular, the domiciliary respiratory care means a set of treatments for patients with breathing problems at their own home. Pulmonologist or critical care patients require this kind of treatment of COPD, and other illness such as chronic bronchitis and emphysema for the lungs in which the airways become narrowed; this leads to a limitation of the flow of air to and from the lungs causing shortness of breath. Other respiratory problems can be side effects of cancer of the larynx. For instance, one of the patients considered for our study presents a chronic bronchitis complicated with a larynx cancer. Other common respiratory problems are asthma, pneumonia (bacterial, viral and chemical ones), collapsed lungs, emphysema, hyperventilation, pleurisy, pulmonary edema, pulmonary embolism etc.

The domiciliary solutions are suitable and much extended in the public health systems, such as those found in Spain, where the public health system rents the systems to third parties. However, the problem continues partially, since only the 42% of the patients, who receive this therapy, satisfy at least the 80% of the therapy prescribed by the pulmonologist. Therefore, the patient needs to be controlled to reach more powerful effect in the patient recovery and health status. Usually the patients with respiratory failure, who do not follow the treatment in a suitable way, are used to living with little oxygen, assuming as usual the breathlessness and tiredness. But they do not understand that is making more difficult that organs such as the heart recover from their illness, and that patients who comply with the treatment are noticing improvements. Finally, the patients need to receive additional treatments such as remove respiratory secretions (e.g. mucus) and clear airway to optimize respiratory function, which are ancillary to the oxygen therapy, such as presented in the Fig. 1.

Therefore, the AAL solutions permit to carry out the treatments for the mentioned patients in their houses, instead of the hospital. Thereby, this improves the quality of life for these patients and reducing the healthcare costs (especially for public health systems as that found in Spain). In case of that these AAL were not defined, these patients in risk, should stay in the hospital full time, in order to be alive.

The current solutions defined for the incorporation of home respiratory therapies, for patients with breathing problems such as the mentioned COPD, have not yet addressed the paradigm of predictive models applied in this environment.

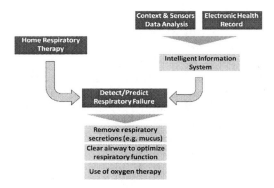

Fig. 1. Therapy model proposed in the AIRE project

Such as presented in Fig. 1, our model is based on the relationship between the levels of oxygen saturation and respiratory rate with their lung capacity, in order to try to predict that before respiratory failure with the goal of clearing respiratory via, removing mucus and apply oxygen therapy. In addition, it can be determinated to carry out an analysis with a spirometer, in order to get more information, which can be used for the Intelligent Information System to determinate whether the anomaly was caused only by an obstruction of the respiratory secretions, or it is a major problem, which can conclude in serious symptoms such as insufficiency respiratory.

During the continuous monitoring, the wearable sensors analyses are focused on detecting simple symptoms such as shortness of breath (i.e. dyspnea) with the breath amplitude sensors, which is one of the most common symptoms of several respiratory diseases such as emphysema, bronchitis and pleurisy. Other symptom considered is hyperventilation with the breath frequency, which can also occur as a consequence of various lung diseases, head injury, or stroke (central neurogenic hyperventilation, apneustic respirations, ataxic respiration, Cheyne-Stokes respirations or Biot's respiration). In addition, it is considered the oxygen saturation (i.e. SpO2), which is highly relevant to detect the insufficiency respiratory, such as presented in one of our previous works [6]. Finally, it is considered the temperature, which is one of the most relevant parameters used for COPD diagnosis, pleurisy and several of the respiratory diseases, which manifest fever. The ongoing work is considering noise sensors to detect wheezing and cough [7].

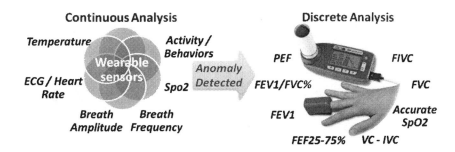

Fig. 2. Relationship between continuous monitoring and the discrete analysis for tele-diagnosis

The continuous monitoring of these parameters is clinically relevant, since some illness such as emphysema usually develops slowly. Patients may not have any acute episodes of shortness of breath. Slow deterioration is the rule, and it may go unnoticed. In addition, after that the patient has been diagnosed, this continuous and real time analysis of the patient allows to detect anomalies, which can ask for some actions to the patient, such as check his current status with some additional sensors such as the spirometer (which offer a higher and accurate quantity of information, which allows to the system the verification of the detected anomaly), ask for the caregivers to clean the respiratory via in case of illness such as larynx cancer, where is required to take out the mucus and apply the oxygen therapy, or ask external attendance in the worst case.

The additional sensors considered in our solution, is a spirometer, which cannot be used continuously, since it needs that the patient must sit up straight, feet flat against the floor and head facing forward in order to get a valid measure. Spirometry has been chosen, since it is the most common test used to evaluate how well the lungs are functioning. Specifically, spirometry measures how quickly air moves in and out of the lungs, and measure the volume and speed of air. This offers several values, such as presented in the Fig. 2. Some of them are very relevant to detect earlier obstructions such as FEF25-75% [8-9]. The current status of the Intelligent Information System is work in progress. For that reason, it is not presented detailed in this paper.

Fig. 3 presents the general view of the home respiratory therapy solution, where are defined different kinds of continuous signals through a wearable system and discrete signals, which as monitored periodically or when an anomaly (i.e. alarm) is detected. The next section is going to present the sensors considered and the platform, to make feasible this home respiratory therapy.

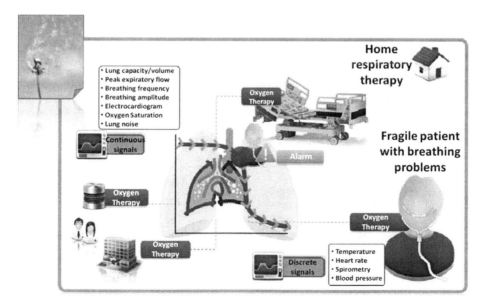

Fig. 3. Home respiratory architecture proposed

3 Home Respiratory Architecture Proposed

The architecture proposed integrates the required sensors involved in the home respiratory therapy in a platform, which allows to communicate the sensors installed in the domiciliary for telemedicine purpose such as the spirometer, and the worn sensors by the patient for continuous monitoring with the Hospital Information System, Intelligent Information Systems, operation managements and remote monitoring centers, such as presented in the Fig. 4.

This kind of solution, for the integration of clinical environment (ICE) at the patient's home can be classified in two levels of solutions. The first level, ICE1, is focused on the safety, which is the level where is found our current work. This level solves the issues such as ensure the integrity, reliability and accurate of the monitored information, interoperability of all the sensors with the platform, and functions to detect fault of the sensors i.e. self-monitoring and healing, auto-configuration, remote management, and finally integration with the second level, ICE, which is focused on clinical decision support, control loops clinical practice guideline conformance, revenue coding for episodes of clinical care.

On the one hand, in order to support the first level, ICE1, it has been defined smart adaptors for the sensors which permit to verify the integrity of the system, protect the data and carry out management tasks. On the other hand, in order to support the second level, ICE2, it is going to be defined by the Intelligent Information System which will manage the information generated by the sensors to detect the respiratory failures, verify continuously the patient status and alarm to caregivers. This second level is being carried out in the ongoing work, such as mentioned in the Section 2.

Our solution to define the ICE1 solution for this scenario is based on Internet of Things, which allows to connect all the devices around the patient such as sensors, and collecting context information such as patient's activity.

The problems found to make feasible the ICE1 with the defined adaptors based on Internet of Things, which in order to reach a low cost, low power consumption, and reduced size, they present a low performance, reduced capacity and resources. Therefore, a set of challenges are defined to offer all the requirements of an ICE1, security and protection of the information, and adaptation to the changes of patients' position, i.e. mobility support. The support for the mobility of the patients have been solved, with a novel mobility protocol, which has been designed to support mobile monitoring of patients and workers for AAL environments, hospitals and critical environments such as refineries [10]. On the other hand, this has been defined an advanced implementation of security based on public key cryptography, which allows the protection of the information end-to-end [11], since the privacy is one of the most relevant issues in healthcare domain.

The system has been designed to work with sensors for medical purpose from different vendors. Therefore, this system has a very flexible and open connectivity support. Specifically are supported medical sensors via RS232 (serial communication) and Bluetooth. But additionally, under this project we are adapting medical sensors to 6LoWPAN, it is a protocol defined by the Internet Engineering Task Force (IETF), which extends Wireless Sensor Networks (WSN) to Internet, adding to IEEE 802.15.4 a layer to support IPv6. 6LoWPAN presents advantages with respect to previous versions of AAL solutions based on Bluetooth, because with 6LoWPAN the value is transmitted directly without user interaction, i.e. user does not need to set up a mobile phone or similar. That feature is very interesting for elderly patients, who are not very used to new technologies, and since COPD is very frequent in elderly population, it is a relevant feature.

The initial step to define this platform has been to determinate the sensors and biomedical devices for monitoring the reduction in breathing capacity, in order to satisfy the therapy presented in the section 2 and Fig. 3. The sensors considered have been, see table 1:

Table 1. Sensors considered for the solution

Sensor	Communication interface	Parameters measured
A&D UA767PC	Serial	Blood Pressure
Nonin WristOx2 3150	Bluetooth	SPo2 and heart rate
Medlab EG00352	Serial (Wearable)	SPo2 and heart rate
CardioBlue MediTech	Bluetooth (Wearable)	Electrocardiogram
Medlab EG01000	Serial (Wearable)	Electrocardiogram
MIR Spirobank II	Serial	PEF; FEV1; FVC; FEF; SPO2
Medlab EG00700	Serial (Wearable)	Temperature
Avita TS-28BT	Bluetooth	Temperature
Asma-1 Vitalograph	USB	PEF; FEV1

The selected biomedical sensors are being adapted to the developed personal device, presented in [12], where previously glucometers from different vendors were connected to a common adaptor with wireless Internet connectivity, in order connect wireless to the AAL gateway developed and presented previously in [13], this has been extended with the Bluetooth transceiver WT12 from Bluegiga, which supports Health Device Profile (HDP) in the 3.1.0 build 385 of the iWrap operating system, HDP is the profile defined by the Continua Alliance and the standard IEEE 1073 for the communication with clinical sensors based on Bluetooth sensors.

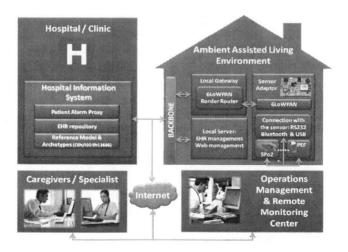

Fig. 4. Integration of the sensors in the platform

The wireless connectivity allows to the patients be monitored at the same time that they carry out their usual activities, the denominated activities daily living (ADL), the wearable sensors are the considered for continuous monitoring, and the selected for this purpose have been those offered by medlab, which allows the easy integration with the developed adaptor, through a simple serial communication.

4   Conclusions and Future Work

The proposed solution goal is to introduce technological innovations and advanced services in the home respiratory therapy to allow patient monitoring and supervision remotely by monitoring centers and the inclusion of intelligent systems to detect the respiratory failure in home therapies, supervising the patient's compliance and alert when the lung capacity from the patient is being reduced. The ongoing work is to define end the definition of the intelligent system to detect the anomalies, and the future work is focused on the integration of the sensors and platform in an orthopedic bed, for patients who are suffering immobility, and the evaluation of the solution in 20 patients with breathing problems in Hospital "Mutua de Terrassa" in Barcelona.

Acknowledgments. This work has been carried out with funds from an award from the Fundación Séneca (04552/GERM/06), the project from the Spanish Ministry for Industry, Tourism and Infrastructure (TSI-020302-2010-95), and the Spanish Ministry of Science and Education with the FPU program grant (AP2009-3981).

References

1. Jaana, M., Paré, G., Sicotte, C.: Home Telemonitoring for Respiratory Conditions: A Systematic Review. The American Journal of Medical Care, 313–320 (May 2009)
2. Bergma, D.: Medic4All Medic4all's telemedicine solution was chosen by the Gertner Institute and Clalit Health Services to operate the largest COPD telemonitoring project in Israel, http://en.medic4all.it/index.php (last access March 2011)
3. Bosch Healthcare, Health Buddy Monitor, http://www.healthbuddy.com and http://www.bosch-telehealth.com (last access March 2011)
4. Trappenburg, J.C.A., Niesink, A., et al.: Effects of Telemonitoring in Patients with Chronic Obstructive Pulmonary Disease. J. Telemedicine and e-Health 14(2), 138–146 (2008)
5. World Health Organization (WHO).: Factsheet about chronic obstructive pulmonary disease (COPD), http://www.who.int/mediacentre/factsheets/fs315/en/index.html (last access March 2011)
6. Jara, A.J., Blaya, F.J., Zamora, M.A., Skarmeta, A.F.G.: An Ontology and Rule Based Intelligent System to Detect and Predict Myocardial Diseases. In: 9th IEEE EMBS Int. Conf. on Information Technology and Applications in Biomedicine, Larnaca, Cyprus (2009)
7. Simpson, C.R., et al.: Trends in the epidemiology of chronic obstructive pulmonary disease in England: a national study of 51804 patients. Brit. J. Gen. Pract. 60(576), 483–488 (2010)

8. Mallett, J., Dougherty, L.: The Royal Marsden Hospital Manual of Clinical Nursing Procedures, 6th edn. Blackwell Science, Oxford (2004)
9. Field, D.: Respiratory care. In: Sheppard, M., Wright, M. (eds.) Principles and Practice of High Dependency Nursing. Baillière Tindall, Edinburgh (2000)
10. Jara, A.J., Silva, R.M., Silva, J.S., Zamora, M.A., Skarmeta, A.F.G.: Mobility IP-based Protocol for Wireless Personal Networks in Critical Environments. In: Wireless Personal Communications. Springer, Heidelberg (2010) (in press)
11. Ayuso, J., Marin, L., Jara, A.J., Skarmeta, A.F.G.: Optimization of Public Key Cryptography (RSA and ECC) for 8-bits Devices based on 6LoWPAN. In: 1st International Workshop on the Security of the Internet of Things (SecIoT 2010), Tokyo, Japan (2010)
12. Jara, A.J., Zamora, M.A., Skarmeta, A.F.G.: An internet of things–based personal device for diabetes therapy management in ambient assisted living (AAL). In: Personal and Ubiquitous Computing (2011) (to be published), doi:10.1007/s00779-010-0353-1
13. Jara, A.J., Zamora, M.A., Skarmeta, A.F.G.: An Architecture for Ambient Assisted Living and Health Environments. In: Omatu, S., Rocha, M.P., Bravo, J., Fernández, F., Corchado, E., Bustillo, A., Corchado, J.M. (eds.) IWANN 2009. LNCS, vol. 5518, pp. 882–889. Springer, Heidelberg (2009)

A 6LoWPAN-Based Foundation for AAL-Applications

Matthias Felsche, Lars Schulz, Andrea Schuster, and Horst Schwetlick

HTW Berlin, Wilhelminenhofstr. 75A, 12459 Berlin, Germany
matthias.felsche@student.htw-berlin.de
lars-manuel.schulz@fhtw-berlin.de
{andrea.schuster,schwetlick}@htw-berlin.de

Abstract. This paper reviews a set of standardized communication technologies, IEEE 802.15.4 and 6LoWPAN for Ambient Assisted Living (AAL). These technologies form a well suited communication stack for applications in this field, enabling body near communication and communication for housing. A sensor/actor network using these standards was implemented on a hardware platform based on the TI CC2430 chip at the wireless lab at the HTW-Berlin (University of Applied Sciences). It is currently coupled with sensors and signal processing for monitoring vital parameters. Results of these developments will support the research in AAL as well as teaching in a new master degree course as an interdisciplinary project between two Berlin Universities (Alice Salomon Hochschule and HTW Berlin) in order to create the next generation products for Ambient Assisted Living (AAL).

1   Introduction

Technical applications for Ambient Assisted Living (AAL) can promote a self-determined live especially for people who can hardly be left alone. The equipment, hardware, and administration of these applications should be as unobtrusive as possible. This requires that the burden of steady surveillance by caring for people shall not be replaced by the struggle of dealing with difficult operation of devices, handling cables, regularly recharging batteries or the pitfalls of a surveillance-system. Therefore it is of an utmost importance to deploy application-systems that are

- fault tolerant and highly available
- unobtrusive
- small and cheap
- able to run for years without intervenience
- if necessary equipped with a very simple and intuitive user interface.

For these development directions in AAL wireless communications serves as an important basis technology. Especially AAL-specific monitoring requires to meet these criteria using a minimum amount of power for operation. Wireless connections can be established easily at a body as well as within buildings. Every single device should be able to operate over very long periods (in best cases for years) having a

J. Bravo, R. Hervás, and V. Villarreal (Eds.): IWAAL 2011, LNCS 6693, pp. 131–136, 2011.
© Springer-Verlag Berlin Heidelberg 2011

simple battery as the only power-supply. By establishing a network of interconnected sensors large application systems become possible.

This paper presents results of ongoing research-activities for wireless platforms and protocols applicable for AAL-scenarios and describes the realized wireless sensor network at the HTW. The important features of IEEE 802.15.4, the protocol stack 6LoWPAN, as well as the operation system FreeRTOS[1] are discussed with respect to AAL applications.

1.1 IEEE 802.15.4

The IEEE 802.15.4 is a standard[2] which is defined for low-rate wireless personal area networks (LR-WPANs) with a range from 10 to 100 meter. The protocol specifies the physical layer and medium access control, which are the lowest two layers of the OSI model. Different protocols for the higher layers are in use, e.g. Zigbee, 6LowPAN and WirelessHART. The system uses the frequencies of industrial, scientific and medical bands (ISM) for operation. These are the unlicensed frequencies in the 868 MHz band in Europe, the 915 MHz in North America and the international band on 2.5 GHz.

The physical layer performs different modulation for a robust wireless communication. One method is the Direct Sequence Spread Spectrum (DSSS) which reduces the susceptibility of the channel. An alternative option is the ASK technique defined for the 868 MHz and 915 MHz frequency band and the Offset Quadrature Phase Shift Keying (O-QPSK). One of the important characteristics of the IEEE 802.15.4 standard is the small packet size of 127 Bytes. This is enough to control a network and to transmit sensor data to an access point (drain). Moreover the transfer rate reaches from 20 kbit/s to 250 kbit/s depending on the used frequency band.

The MAC layer supports two modes of operation. At first a beacon mode using Time Division Multiple Access (TDMA) which guarantees time slots to network-participants and handles node association. These beacons are sent by the coordinator that is for example an access point, to inform the clients about the Contention-Access-Period (CAP), the Contention-Free-Period (CFP) and the Inactive Period of the network. The Inactive Period defines a timeslot in that the nodes can power off. The alternative to the beacon mode is the Carrier Sense Multiple Access (CSMA) to allocate the wireless channel.

```
  0                   1                   2                   3
  0 1 2 3 4 5 6 7 0 1 2 3 4 5 6 7 0 1 2 3 4 5 6 7 0 1 2 3 4 5 6 7
 +-+-+-+-+-+-+-+-+-+-+-+-+-+-+-+-+-+-+-+-+-+-+-+-+-+-+-+-+-+-+-+-+
 |_|Frame-Length |_|C|A|P|S|ftype|SAM|FV |DAM|_|_| Sequence     |
 +-+-+-+-+-+-+-+-+-+-+-+-+-+-+-+-+-+-+-+-+-+-+-+-+-+-+-+-+-+-+-+-+
 |          Addressing Fields - 4 to 20 Octets              ... |
 +-+-+-+-+-+-+-+-+-+-+-+-+-+-+-+-+-+-+-+-+-+-+-+-+-+-+-+-+-+-+-+-+
 |      Auxiliary Security Header 0,5,6,10 or 14 Octets     ... |
 +-+-+-+-+-+-+-+-+-+-+-+-+-+-+-+-+-+-+-+-+-+-+-+-+-+-+-+-+-+-+-+-+
 |                      Data Payload                        ... |
 +-+-+-+-+-+-+-+-+-+-+-+-+-+-+-+-+-+-+-+-+-+-+-+-+-+-+-+-+-+-+-+-+
 | Frame Check Sequence (CRC)  |
 +-+-+-+-+-+-+-+-+-+-+-+-+-+-+-+-+
```

Fig. 1. Schematic view of IEEE 802.15.4 Data-Frame and PHY-Packet

---

[1] http://www.freertos.org/
[2] [IEEE802.15.4].

Furthermore the MAC header (see figure 1) contains the destination and source address and the PAN address. The address size is 16 or 64 Bit, enough for every node in a network to have a unique identification number.

Transceiver chips for the IEEE 802.15.4 supports Interfaces to add Sensors for example to equip the processing unit with acceleration sensors or a voice transmission to observe when an elder people needs some help [WSAN-AAL]. Another advantage of the IEEE 802.15.4 radio Transceiver chips is the adjustment of the transmission power in a range of 25 dB [CC2430]. In a Body Area Network(BAN) it is not necessary to send with the maximum power of 0dBm which is equivalent to 1 mW. Transceiver chips close to each other could send with a reduced transmit power. A decrease of the Transmission power of 25dB is equivalent to 3,2 µW. This conserves battery lifetime and may reduce fears and concerns towards wireless applications and electromagnetic radiation.

1.2 6LoWPAN

Several Network stacks are based on IEEE 802.15.4. Among them the Z-stack, a Zig-Bee-conform network stack by TI[3], WirelessHart and MiWi. We considered 6LoWPAN for our network-stack because it is an open IETF-standard whose implementations entails less overhead than for example the ZigBee-stack.

The 6LoWPAN standard consists of a number of RFCs and Internet Drafts[4] worked out by the Internet Engineering Task Force (IETF) Working Group called 6LoWPAN. This standard defines a compressed IPv6-based network-layer above IEEE 802.15.4 conform devices. The whole stack is shown in figure 2. The Internet Control Message Protocol version 6 is used in 6LoWPAN for establishing and maintaining the PAN. Usually 6LoWPAN is used together with UDP as a minimal Transport Layer which is compressed to.

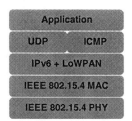

Fig. 2. 6LoWPAN Protocol Stack

6LoWPAN networks are usually stub networks that consist of tiny embedded devices connected to the outer IPv6 internet by a border router which performs the necessary compression and decompression of data-packets from and to the PAN.

An IEEE 802.15.4 Frame has a maximum size of 127 Bytes and in worst case there are only 72 Bytes left for the MPDU. 6LoWPAN Header Compression[5] makes it

---

[3] http://focus.ti.com/docs/toolsw/folders/print/z-stack.html
[4] As defined in [RFC4919] and [RFC4944] and further additional internet-drafts.
[5] See [RFC4944].

possible to shrink a usual IPv6/UDP-header with around 48 Bytes in size to at best 6 Bytes by leaving out redundant data that is given by the context, see figure 3. So there is (at best) 108 Byte space for application-payload. If packets do not fit at all, they can be fragmented.[6]

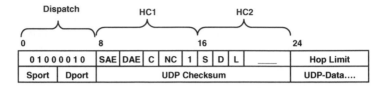

Fig. 3. Compressed 6LoWPAN-Header and UDP-Header

By now there is no standardized way of routing in 6LoWPAN, partly because routing is a problem apart from the main tasks of the 6LoWPAN working group. In 2008 a new working group called *Routing Over Low-power and Lossy networks (ROLL)* was founded to deal with that topic in particular. Their protocol called *IPv6 Routing Protocol for Low power and Lossy Networks (RPL)*[7] exists in its 17th version and is currently under evaluation by the IESG to become an internet standard.

As sensor networks can scale from tens to thousands of nodes and memory and computing resources are very rare, a routing protocol has to scale with reasonable slope.[8] RPL establishes a Distance Oriented Directed Acyclic Graph (DODAG) rooted at the border router as topology to facilitate routing in a hierarchical fashion.

Simulations[9] with a network-setup of 45 nodes have shown that 90% of all nodes need to store less than 10 nodes in their routing tables and that routing control traffic is negligible in respect to the data-traffic-rate.

The self-organization and networking-capabilities of the 6LoWPAN protocol are ideal for an AAL application. A 6LoWPAN-node automatically connects to a gateway and without an intervention by the user (elderly or disable people) or an administrator. The connectivity provided by a 6LoWPAN edge router allows the direct connection to the internet. Massages from the local 6LoWPAN network could inform other services over the internet. For example an emergency-center could be called when it comes to irregularities in a patients physical condition.

1.3 Operating Systems and Hardware Platforms

The described stack is available on a variety of operating systems specialized on embedded devices and sensor networks. In our development and testing network (see figure 4 for a network node) we run the 6LoWPAN-Nanostack 1.1.0 on top of FreeRTOS. But there are several other 6LoWPAN stacks available on TinyOS, Contiki and many more. It has been adapted by the ZigBee Foundation, too.

---

[6] See [ShelbyBormann2009].
[7] As defined in [ROLL-RPL] and other related drafts and RFCs (http://datatracker.ietf.org/wg/roll/)
[8] RPL specific requirements defined in [RPL-Requirements].
[9] See [RPL-Simulation].

This stack is available for all hardware platforms that are supported by the operating systems running a 6LoWPAN-stack over IEEE 802.15.4. Furthermore the operating systems support the connection of sensors and processing of the sensor data on the microprocessor.

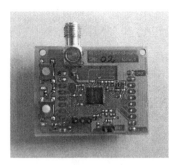

Fig. 4. Radio Engineering Group - 6LoWPAN-development board based on the TI CC2430SoC

1.4   Applications

The entire wireless system for AAL monitoring-applications contains the Version 1.1.0 of FreeRTOS, 6LoWPAN and IEEE 802.15.4 (2006). 6LoWPAN allows to be connected to the local subnet or the whole internet, be it IPv6 or IPv4[10]. Furthermore every single node is reachable and addressable. The whole PAN can get configured and bootstrapped automatically. Remote configuration and maintenance is possible. It can be seamlessly integrated into existing infrastructures. This system is highly robust and scalable so nearly every reasonable size of application or network is possible.

The system, designed for the usage for Wireless Personal Area Networks serves in Body Area Networks as well. In this respect it supports monitoring applications in health care, wellness and sports. Regarding the usual size of a node it is aspired to embed it into clothing. Different sensors for vital parameters as blood pressure, skin resistance, heart beat or even EEG are connectable to the nodes. This integration including the integrated signal processing and evaluation of the measured data, running on the microcomputer of the sensor nodes is current research at the Radio Engineering Group at the HTW, particular the evaluation of the acoustic heart beat [HeartSound1997]. The used chip (CC2430) with the 6LoWPAN-stack supports conversion of audio signals with a resolution up to 12 bits and a sample rate of 8 kHz.[11] Actual results will be presented in the oral presentation.

These topics will play a significant role within the AAL activities at HTW Berlin, not only in research but in an emerging four semester AAL-master-program. This modular program is for engineers, social educators and designers with a bachelor or diploma degree. It includes interdisciplinary Projects and Design-Thinking for students joining their different backgrounds to develop new perspectives while getting in touch with real application scenarios e.g. elder people and her requirements. It will enable the AAL-students to create ancillary equipment for elderly people, since sensor networks are one basis to support social communities, work, mobility and

---

[10] Which is reachable via IPv6-in IPv4-tunneling.
[11] See [CC2430].

monitoring systems in the field of AAL. It is a great step forward to teach current state-of-the-art in sensor networks, future directions and research challenges in developing and deploying sensor networks and other technologies, e.g. body sensor networks and wireless sensor networks in the context of AAL.

1.5 Summary

In this paper a wireless system with a standardized network protocol-stack has been presented as a powerful foundation for AAL-applications. Its huge capabilities have rendered it fully applicable for sensoring- and monitoring-based applications like surveillance of vital-functions, position-tracking, etc. The wireless system supports different research in AAL-projects at the HTW. The results and experiences lead to the development of a new master degree course with main focus on AAL.

References

[RFC4919] Kushalnagar, N., Montenegro, G., Schumacher, C.: IPv6 over Low-Power Wireless Personal Area Networks (6LoWPANs): Overview, Assumptions, Problem State-ment, and Goals. RFC 4919 (informational) (August 2007),
http://www.ietf.org/rfc/rfc4919.txt

[RFC4944] Montenegro, G., Kushalnagar, N., Hui, J., Culler, D.: Transmission of IPv6 Packets over IEEE 802.15.4 Networks. RFC 4944 Proposed Standard (September 2007),
http://www.ietf.org/rfc/rfc4944.txt

[IEEE802.15.4] IEEE: Wireless Medium Access Control (MAC) and Physical Layer (PHY) Specifications for Low-Rate Wireless Personal Area Networks (WPANs), IEEE 802.15.4-2006 (September 2006)

[ROLL-RPL] Winter, T., Thubert, P., et al.: Pv6 Routing Protocol for Low power and Lossy Networks. draft-ietf-roll-rpl-14, Internet Draft (December 2010),
http://www.ietf.org/internet-drafts/draft-ietf-roll-rpl-17.txt

[RPL-Requirements] Levis, P., Tavakoli, A., Dawson-Haggerty, S.: Overview of Exist-ing Routing Protocols for Low Power and Lossy Networks, draft-ietf-roll-protocols-survey-07, Internet Draft (April 2009), http://tools.ietf.org/html/draft-ietf-roll-protocols-survey-07

[RPL-Simulation] Tripathi, J., et al.: Performance Evaluation of Routing Protocol for Low-Power and Lossy Networks (RPL). draft-tripathi-roll-rpl-simulation-04, Internet-Draft (Juni 2010),
http://www.ietf.org/id/draft-tripathi-roll-rpl-simulation-04.txt

[KuprisSikora2007] Kupris, G., Sikora, A.: Zigbee Datenfunk im IEEE 802.15.4. Franzis Verlag, Poing (2007)

[ShelbyBormann2009] Shelby, Z., Bormann, C.: 6LoWPAN. In: The Wireless Embedded Internet. Wiley Series on Communications Networking & Distributed Systems. Wiley, Chichester (2009)

[HeartSound1997] Liang, H., Lukkarinen, S., Hartimo, I.: Heart sound segmentation algorithm based on heart sound envelogram. In: Computers in Cardiology 1997, Lund, Sweden, pp. 105–108 (1997)

[CC2430] CC2430 Datasheet: A true System-on-Chip solution for 2.4 GHz IEEE802.15.4/ZigBee. Texas Instruments Incorporated (2009)

[WSAN-AAL] Delicato, F.C., Fuentes, L., Gámez, N., Pires, P.F.: Variabilities of wireless and actuators sensor network middleware for ambient assisted living. In: Omatu, S., Rocha, M.P., Bravo, J., Fernández, F., Corchado, E., Bustillo, A., Corchado, J.M. (eds.) IWANN 2009. LNCS, vol. 5518, pp. 851–858. Springer, Heidelberg (2009)

SENIORCHANNEL
An Interactive Digital Television Channel for Promoting Entertainment and Social Interaction amongst Elderly People

Ana Hernandez[1], Francisco Ibañez[2], and Neftis Atallah[3]

[1] Indra Software Labs, Acanto 11,
28045 Madrid, Spain
[2] Brainstrom Multimedia, Maestro Gozalbo 23,
46005 Valencia Spain
[3] Cedetel, Parque Tecnológico de Boecillo,
47151 Boecillo, Valladolid, Spain
ahernandezma@indra.es, francisco@brainstorm.es,
tneftis@cedetel.es

Abstract. SeniorChannel is a project funded under call 2 of Ambient Assisted Living Program AAL, whose objective is the development of an Interactive Internet Protocol Television Channel (SENIORCHANNEL) that will not only provide elderly people with a method of interacting but also with a unique means of access to the range of diverse activities in their community including the opportunity to share knowledge and experience, the ability to participate in topical debates, entertainment services, work-shops and discussion groups regardless of their geographical location. Also will be developed and implemented a low cost, easy-to-use, integrated TV studio and production centre that will enable community driven broadcasting.

Keywords: Social TV, Elderly People, Interactive TV.

1 Project Overview

The project SeniorChannel is funded under call 2 of Ambient Assisted Living Program (AAL) and has a budget of 4.329.045 € of which 2.0 million Euros is provided by the AAL Joint Programme.

SeniorChannel is a 3 year project leaded by Indra Software Labs and brings together 11 partners and subcontractors from five different European countries involving one university: University of Padova, five Small Enterprise: Brainstorm, Audemat, WinMedia, WhiteLoop, M31 and Innovatec, one Research Centre: Cedetel, one Industrial partner: Indra Software Labs and two User's Centres: Asociacion Parque Galicia and Linköpings Kommun.

The vision in project SeniorChannel is based on the assumption that the quality of life for elderly people in our communities will be improved if advanced network technologies can be used to facilitate engagement and interaction amongst them, both

J. Bravo, R. Hervás, and V. Villarreal (Eds.): IWAAL 2011, LNCS 6693, pp. 137–142, 2011.

directly and indirectly. As people get older, their roles in life and the community change.

They retire from professional life and relinquish the responsibility that comes with parenthood; this can lead to disengagement as they feel their involvement in society is less valued compared to when they were younger and more active.

The goal in project SeniorChannel is to integrate innovative technologies and high added value content in order to provide elderly people with an opportunity to interact and share their knowledge, opinions and aspirations with the wider community and derive enjoyment from the experience.

Furthermore, SeniorChannel will give elderly care professionals an innovative approach to developing and managing the specific social needs of the elderly in the wider community.

To achieve this goal, SeniorChannel will develop an Interactive Internet Protocol Television Channel (SENIORCHANNEL) that will not only provide elderly people with a method of interacting but also with a unique means of access to the range of diverse activities in their community including the opportunity to share knowledge and experience, the ability to participate in topical debates, entertainment services, work-shops and discussion groups regardless of their geographical location.

The unique approach to be adopted by the SeniorChannel consortium is to develop and implement a low cost, easy-to-use, integrated TV studio and production centre that will enable community driven broadcasting. SeniorChannel will also provide new business opportunities through direct access to a growing segment in the market.

The SeniorChannel technology will facilitate interaction between elderly people themselves, as well as others for whom the elderly person's well-being is of particular interest, such as, care supervisors and the family of the elderly person. This will be of particular use in situations where elderly people are geographically dispersed.

The technology developed in this project consist in a integrated TV studio and production centre, installed at the Users Centres and a STB specially adapted for this project installed in the elderly person's home. For both developments the user's requirements collected from the users and care supervisor of the Users Centres will be an essential point of reference.

Historically the TV has been a passive media, but digital television has made new services possible which the user can access easily without more difficult. SENIORCHANNEL will integrate robust and reliable interfacing technologies based on hybrid DTT and IPTV STB (Set-top Box) that facilitate the interaction of elderly people with outside world through the TV. Simply using a Set Top Box and a TV remote control device, specifically selected for the project, the elderly people will be able to access at home to a wide range of interactive services: information services as weather forecast, communication services as chat, entertainment services, health services,... Besides, the developed channel in the project will introduce a higher interactivity by allowing end users to communicate with the TV program presenters thanks to the videoconference capacity of the system. Webcams in the houses of the user will be connected to digital decoders (STB) to support this functionality.

At the TV production site a low cost integrated TV studio and production centre will be created integrating real time video and graphics applications that allow the production and broadcast of high quality interactive programmes. In addition a bidirectional information system will be developed to manage all the contents to be displayed on the TV and the interactive information coming from elderly people at their place of residence. This information which will include for example option selection and video stream from the webcams will enable programs to be conducted according to the opinions and preferences of elderly people in real time. The webcam at users' sites will also provide users at home with the opportunity to participate in debates integrating the image in the TV general video stream and offering the audience the possibility of associating a voice to a face and so get to know each other in a virtual way.

2 Project Status

In the first annually the collecting phase of user's requirement has been carried out, leaded by University of Padova. It have been performed several studios about the behaviour and necessities of elderly people as well as a design guidelines for the development of Interactive TV applications oriented to older users which will help in the next development stage.

The protocols for interviewing the final users about their preference for system functionalities and content were designed. Using this methodology a consultation event was celebrated at the user's centre Asociación Parque Galicia which was focused on identifying specific types of activities that would be both enjoyable and of practical valued. The result of this consultation was the guide for the specification process of Users Requirements.

In this annuity the global architecture for the SeniorChannel System has been defined. This architecture is formed by:

- Virtual TV Studio to produce TV Programs to be broadcasted on-line. It will be installed at the user's Center.
- STB at user's homes to access to on-line TV programs or on-demand content
- A Multimedia Data Base to store on-demand content. All the on-line programs will be stored in the Data Base once its have been broadcasted.
- A play-out server to process the video streaming.
- A web-server to process the data interchange between the other components of the system.

One of the most important developments in SeniorChannel Project is the setting up of a Virtual Studio to produce TV Programs in the Senior Centres without investing in expensive physical sets. With only a fixed camera, a video mixer and a chromakey, the centres will be able to produce their own programs in a very attractive virtual set with advanced 3D graphics that will add realism to the live or recorded programs to broadcast. In this research field, Brainstorm Multimedia has developed a low cost virtual studio software that integrates the video mixer and the chromakey in the own software. Besides, the company is developing a software application that allows designing and creating full 3D virtual studio scene very quickly with no prior experience. We think that active elderly people will be able to use it and create different sets for the programs to be produced and developed by them. In this

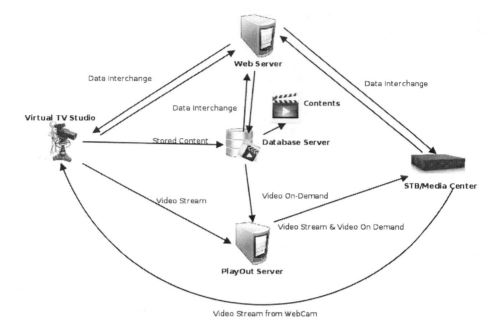

Fig. 1. SeniorChannel Architecture

software, a simple and intuitive interface allows the user to select from a library of pre-defined backgrounds, floors, wall and furniture. The objects within the 3D set can then be coloured, textured and positioned in full 3D space as required. Once the camera position is chosen, the output is then fed to the chromakey for compositing of the foreground image. The application also includes a text generator with simple animations.

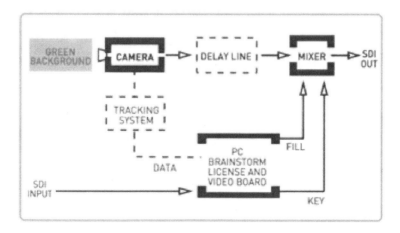

Fig. 2. Virtual TV Studio's Specification System

The application is supported in Windows, Linux and Mac OSX platforms and it is recommended with a PC with the latest microprocessors and video and graphics boards like Bluefish 444, AJA 2Xs, AJA HS/2Ke, and Nvidia Quadro FX5500, FX5600, FX5500SDI and FX5600SDI.

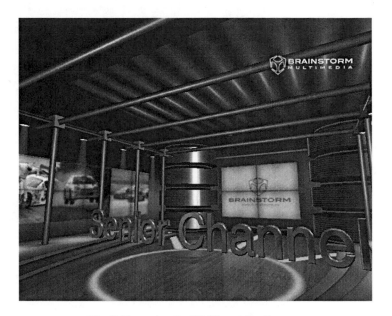

Fig. 3. Example of a 3D Virtual Studio scene

3   Future Developments

Once the SeniorChannel architecture has been defined and the users requirements has been stabilised, the work will be centred in the development and implementation of the low cost TV Studio, an interactive Information System and an intuitive Interaction System.

For Brainstorm, the main future work is to finish the development of the low cost virtual studio, the implementation in the elderly centre and carry out the technical validation producing some standard TV programs with the developed technologies. It will be essential to train the elderly people in the use of the applications specifically designed and developed for an easy and intuitive use. In parallel, software for creating a full 3D virtual scene will be developed and validated with the users. This intuitive software will allow users to compose a 3D virtual set by selecting 3D objects from a library of pre-defined backgrounds, floor, walls, furniture and screens. Different virtual sets will be created for each TV program produced by elderly people and it will be broadcasted in live or recorded and edited for on-demand TV.

Indra Software Labs will develop an interactive Information System based on a Web Server which will control the data interchange between the STB, the Multimedia Data Base and the TV Studio. The Web Server allows the system to be interactive for the users, they will be able to participate in several TV program broadcasted online, answering questions or selecting between several options. These data will be transmitted to the Web Server which will redirect it to the Virtual Studio to include them in the broadcasted signal. Also, the Server will be the link between user's STB and Multimedia Database in order to access to the list of on-demand content available to the user.

The future contributions of CEDETEL in SeniorChannel will focus on development of interactive services compatibles with hybrid IPTV and DTT system. This task includes the design and the development of a collection of applications to add interaction with STB via easy remote control devices, looking for simplicity of use for elderly people. IPTV technology allows to offer videoconferencing capabilities, providing a high interaction in real time among system users and with the presenter located in the TV Studio. The main goal of the platform is to improve the relationship with older people and help to reduce the risk of social exclusion.

4 Conclusions

The main challenge of the project is to train elderly people in the use of all the technology involved in a TV program generation and obtain an IP-TV made for and by elderly people. With the easy to use and intuitive technology developed in the project, the consortium is very confident in the capability of elderly people to work in teams and to cope with the applications to generate TV programs. All the activities related to the development of a TV program will promote the team work and the socialization of elderly people, the main aim of the AAL Programme.

References

1. SeniorChannel website, http://innovation-labs.com/seniorchannel/
2. Ambient Assisted Living Join Programme, http://www.aal-europe.eu/

An Interactive Content Service for Photo Frames in the Home

Carlos Lopes[1], Rui José[1], and Ana Aguiar[2]

[1] University of Minho, Portugal
pg13385@alunos.uminho.pt, rui@dsi.uminho.pt
[2] FEUP, Porto, Portugal
anaa@fe.up.pt

Abstract. In this paper, we describe an approach for enabling digital photo frames to become generic interaction devices for the home. Their off-the-shelf nature and the simplicity of their interaction model can make photo frames a key element in the AAL eco-system. The motivating hypothesis for this work is that an externally managed image feed can be used to display information associated with AAL services. We have conceived and evaluated a content delivery service for off-the-shelf wireless photo frames that enables interaction with remote content using only the standard photo frame controls. Evaluation results have shown that the proposed approach is able to support multiple interaction modes, but they have also highlighted technical challenges associated with cache management in some photo frame models. This work represents a contribution towards enabling photo frames to become building blocks for interactive services in AAL scenarios.

Keywords: Ambient Display, Digital Photo Frame, Interaction, AAL.

1 Introduction

Ambient Assisted Living (AAL) aims to leverage on smart technologies to address the needs of elderly people, enabling a more independent and socially engaging life. AAL technologies have had a particular focus on the home environment, for which numerous technological infrastructures have been proposed as enablers for the intended services. However, the effective deployment and usage of these technologies has been somewhat restrained by the considerable challenges involved in setting up appropriate infrastructures at home and developing the everyday practices to match the potential of those technologies.

An alternative and more organic approach to AAL deployment is to leverage on the increasing availability of off-the-shelf digital devices that are already Internet-enabled and part of people's everyday practices. This may include more personal devices, such as mobile phones, PDAs and MP3 players, but increasingly also others types of networked devices, such as as energy meters, cameras, and digital photo frames. The presence of these networked devices in the home may lead to the emergence of a new home eco-system in which many new interaction

J. Bravo, R. Hervás, and V. Villarreal (Eds.): IWAAL 2011, LNCS 6693, pp. 143–150, 2011.
© Springer-Verlag Berlin Heidelberg 2011

patterns may emerge as appropriate and in which the devices can be integrated with complimentary services to gain entirely new roles with considerable added value. A broad set of rich digital services may thus reach the home this way, rather than through the traditional personal computer interface or some type of dedicated infrastructure.

In this paper, we describe an approach for enabling digital photo frames to become generic interaction devices for the home. Photo frames can be appropriated for entirely new purposes when networked and integrated into a service: they have clearly reached mass market and can now easily be bought anywhere and taken home; they offer a simple and well-known interaction paradigm based on content iteration; and, as interactive displays, they have the potential to support a very vast range of services combining push and pull information modes. Despite being designed to display photo collections, networked photo frame can also be used as part of an external service, in which case those images may no longer be just photos, but any information that is considered relevant at the moment, transforming the photo frame into a generic display for the devices and services of the home. The motivating hypothesis for this work is that a properly managed image feed can be used to support interactive content on a photo frame and that such photo frame could be deployed and operated without requiring much more than the display itself and a wireless connection. This approach may be especially appealing to AAL scenarios, given the target population and the nature of many of the proposed services. We can observe from the AAL literature that many of the envisioned services include some sort of informative purpose or need the ability to generate notifications to the people living in the Home. With this approach, such functionality could be achieved by simply buying an off-the-shelf photo frame and allowing the various AAL services in the Home to expose their content through the photo frame service using standard web technologies.

We have conceived and evaluated a content delivery service for off-the-shelf wireless photo frames that enables interaction with remote content using only the standard photo frame controls. Evaluation results have shown that it is possible to support multiple interaction modes, although it has also highlighted technical challenges associated with cache management in some photo frame models.

2   Related Work

The idea of a generic content delivery service for photo frames has already been explored by commercially available services. FrameIt[1] and FrameChannel[2] are examples of services that augment digital photo frames by enabling owners to manage the content that is delivered by the service to the device. Users can select from multiple content sources, such as personal photo collections, local weather, news, financial and local information. Channels can be scheduled so that they are only displayed at a specific time of the day, and they can be given priorities to improve content selection. These services share with our work the

---

[1] http://frameit.live.com/
[2] http://www.framechannel.com/

idea of generating a flexible RSS image feed to present content on photo frames. However, none of these services supports the type of interaction alternatives that we considered to be crucial for most AAL scenarios.

The use of small displays in the home environment has also been explored in multiple ways. The Shoebox [1] project combines the storage and display of digital photos in one single device. The aim was to explore new ways of interacting with digital photos that are similar to the interactions using physical photos, and also to promote methods of storing and interacting with photos that would stimulate the local sharing of photos and stories. The Whereabouts Clock [2] provides awareness about the location of the family elements. It serves mainly as an ambiente display for the home, existing mainly in the periphery of attention, and allowing the family to occasionally glance at the information displayed. The CareNet Display [3] is an augmented digital photo frame designed to help elders' caregivers with information about the everyday life of the elder. The device can be used as an ambient display, but it also supports interactions that enable the members of the care-network of the elder to access more information. In the ambient display mode the CareNet Display shows the overall data of the elder's day, such as if the elder has eaten and other relevant occurrences. The interactive mode enables a deeper inquiry of the elder's daily information, such as at what hours the elder has eaten. This daily information that is shown by the device originates from input by the elder, the caregivers or from sensors that monitor the house. The TxtBoard [4] is a small display that shows the SMS messages that have been sent to it, exploring a person-to-place communication pattern. The prototype was intentionally built as a simple device, underlining its function as a message display. The use of an already existing communication method (the sms) and its peripheral nature, allowed TxtBoard to add value to the home ecosystem without imposing a major changes to the family lifestyle and practices. The HomeNote [5] project extended TxtBoard with the possibility to allow users to scribble notes in the screen using stylus markings. It enabled similar interaction patterns, as those found in the TxtBoard, but the scribble feature added some new types of messaging, such as broadcasting identity, reminders, passing on messages and information store. These projects have provided an important contribution to our work, highlighting many of the communication patterns that can be enabled by this type of small displays and informing our design of a more generic approach. While each of these systems is designed with a particular objective, we aim to explore how to integrate a generic interactive functionality using off-the-shelf digital photo frames.

3 System Overview

We have developed the interactive informative Display (iiD) system to address the challenges of supporting interaction with remote content on off-the-shelf digital photo frames. To inform our design process, we have conducted an extensive study of usage situations for this type of small digital display, including home scenarios in the literature, but also other application domains, such as room reservation displays or ambient displays for the office. In particular, we sought to identify the interaction modes that were needed for an effective interaction model, and we have identified the following three: Push, Pull and Notification.

In the Content Push mode, the display is iterating through a content pool and content is shown without any user intervention. This is the most obvious and common scenario and is already supported by existing services. It will be henceforth referred to as the normal mode. As an additional requirement, the display service should enable content to be selected considering some measure of its current relevance. The system would then be able to select which content items from a potentially large content pool are deemed more appropriate at any given moment based on the content itself or in the context of its presentation.

In the Content Pull mode, the user interacts with the display to request a specific content item. This is not necessarily the ability to request arbitrary content. It may simply correspond to the ability to request a content item from a small content list. Still, a pull model is key in enabling the user to actively seek a specific content item whenever needed.

In the Notification mode, the display locks itself on a single content item until the user explicitly interacts, thus confirming that the presented information has been seen. A variant is the temporary notification mode, which works exactly the same way, except that there is some time limit associated with the notification, after which the photo frame should resume its normal operation mode. This is essentially a feature to support asynchronous communication, allowing people to be informed about relevant events that have occurred when they were not paying attention to the display. For example, a medicine reminder service may post a note about taking the pills, or a new message sent to the display may stay there until the person acknowledges having seen it. A temporary notification may be posted to alert the person for lower priority or transient events, such as an update on the content of one the services.

3.1   Event Model

This work is based on the assumption that a digital photo frame can be configured with the URL of an image feed and that the photo frame will then use HTTP to obtain that feed and each of the individual images referenced in the feed. The photo frame may start iterating through the photos in the feed, but it may also support explicit control of the presentation sequence through interactive controls. The most common form of interaction supported by photo frames is the existence of buttons to switch between photos, allowing the viewer to explicitly move back and forward in the photo sequence. These controls may also be available in the form of a remote control or in a touch-sensitive part of the display, but the essence of the interaction remains the same. We thus chose to base our interaction design solely on these capabilities, in order to guarantee that the proposed approach would be applicable across most photo frame products, regardless of the specificities of their interaction alternatives.

The approach is based on decoupling the back and forward buttons of the photo frames from their traditional iteration semantics. This is achieved by building on top of the HTTP requests generated by the photo frame an event model that supports other interpretations of the user interactions with the photo frame. When the photo frame requests an image feed, it receives a generic feed with N items (where N > 3) in which the urls corresponding to the images are simply indicating numbered names, such a 1.jpg, 2.jpg. and so on. As part of its normal operation mode, the photo frame is configured to iterate through the images every T seconds. Assuming that the photo frame cache is disabled, every change in the displayed image results in a new HTTP request to the server. In its normal iteration model, this will mean that the photo frame will issue an HTTP request for the next image in the sequence after T seconds. However, if the forward or back buttons are used, different request patterns will occur and may be detected by the server to generate the three types of event described in table 1.

Table 1. Requests and Events

HTTP request	Events generated
Previous image in the feed sequence	**Rewind :** This event is interpreted as an indication that the user has pushed the back button.
Next image before **T** seconds	**Forward :** This event is interpreted as an indication that the user has pushed the forward button in the photo frame.
Next image after **T** seconds	**Timed next :** This event is interpreted as part of the normal iteration process when the photo frame automatically requests the next content to be displayed.

Based on these events, we have implemented two types of interactive controls: menus and shortlists. In a menu, the displayed content corresponds to a binary option, with the left option being chosen with the back button and the right option being chosen with the forward button. The menu can have multiple levels and the options will continue until a leaf option is reached. This may result in a deep hierarchy, but a proper distribution of the options should guarantee that the most popular ones are closer to the root of the menu tree. Shortlists are essentially a sequence of selected content, in which specific content items can be quickly iterated using the frame controls. The shortlist is shown as any other feed content, but moving back and forward will iterate through the pre-defined items in the shortlist, rather than any content the server could decide to show next. When in the normal mode, the menu mode can be activated by pushing the back button and the shortlist mode by pushing the forward button.

In addition to the above events, the iiD system also supports the notification events. These events do not originate from the photo frame. They are generated by the content services, which are allowed to generate them in order to trigger notifications related with their own information. These include the Alert and the Temp Alert events. The state diagram described in Fig. 1 represents the various system states and how those events can originate state transitions.

When in the auto mode, the system is iterating through the content, simply returning the next item in the sequence for every TimedNext event. A Rewind

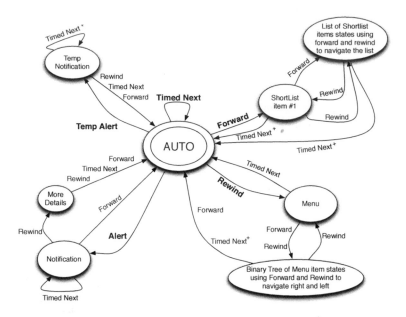

Fig. 1. iiD state diagram

event will move the system into menu mode, making subsequent requests to be interpreted as part of menu interaction. A Forward event will move the system into Shortlist mode, making subsequent requests to be interpreted as part of iterations through the selected items. When a service triggers a notification, the system moves into the Notification or Temp Notification modes. In both cases, new requests that generate a TimedNext event will be answered with the same notification image, thus giving the perception that the frame is locked on that information. The system returns to the Auto mode when a Forward or Rewind event is generated, indicating that a button has been pressed. In the Notification mode, it is also possible to distinguish between a Rewind event, interpreted as a request for further details about the notification, and the Forward event, interpreted as the intention to go back to auto mode. In the TimedNotification, and after the specified validity time has been reached, the system will automatically go back to Auto mode.

4   Evaluation

To validate and gain additional insight into the proposed approach, we have developed a prototype implementation of an interactive service for photo frames, called iiD system, and we have conducted a simple user study to validate the proposed interaction modes.

4.1   Implementation

We have created a web-based implementation of an iiD server using ASP.net technology and a Model-View-Controller pattern [6]. The Controller interprets HTTP requests received from the photo frame, generating the corresponding events and instructing the view and the model to adjust as required. The view runs the presentation of information, which in our case corresponds to the feed that is displayed in the photo frame and the content that gets inserted into the respective images. The data model is composed by a set of content services, each being able to provide information for a particular set of content items. While any web application could be used, the visualization requirements of the small photo frame display lead us to create our own set of simple web applications that could gather the necessary data and display it in an appropriate way. An image creation service was used to take a snapshot of the service content and render it as an image. For the purpose of this prototype we have developed service modules for news, for e-mail, triggering an alert event when there was e-mail to be read, and a Facebook module that cycles through content in a Facebook page and sets a temporary alert event new wall messages are posted.

A potential technical limitation that we have identified with the photo frame we were initially using was that, even with the cache disabled, the device would still use the cached images instead of retrieving the images from the server. While this may not necessarily be the case with other photo frame models, the details of cache management are not normally available in the technical information about photo frames, representing a major obstacle to the selection of devices with the appropriate characteristics. As a consequence, for the purpose of this evaluation we have decided to emulate a photoframe using a touch-screen device.

4.2   User Study

In order to evaluate the concept and particularly its interactive features, we have deployed the display in an administrative office within the University to serve as an Ambient Display for a period of 4 weeks. We have collected usage logs and conducted semi-structured interviews with some of the people working in that space. An initial interview, one week into the experiment, was mainly focused on usability and served to identify minor improvements that were then introduced into the system, such as the overall appeal of the views, the size of text fonts and additional context about content, such as author or date published.

The evaluation setting was clearly not the most appropriate, given the presence of multiple other displays calling for people's attention, but the evaluation results have still shown an overall positive view of the display and its underlying concept. In the final interviews, users have mainly expressed suggestions that were clear improvements to the existing model, but none that would challenge the key features of the system. The main suggestions were the inclusion of information providing a sense of progress through the content list, e.g. "2 of 15" items and facilitating the interaction in the shortlist mode by adding the titles of the contents that will appear if the forward or rewind buttons are pressed.

From the system logs we found that only 1,3% of the deployment time was used in either shortlist or menu modes. These 1,3% are divided in 1% for the shortlist and 0.3% for the menu. Regarding notifications, the time it took for someone to interact with the display after an alert was triggered was, on average, 8 minutes and 39 seconds, which considering the experiment setting may be considered as a signal that people were paying attention to the display content.

5   Conclusion

The iiD system is designed to augment digital photo frames by enabling their standard interactive controls to become interactive features for remote content. This is achieved without any changes to the original digital photo frame firmware, which represents a major opportunity for unleashing photo frames as general purposed displays. Their off-the-shelf nature and the simplicity of their interaction model can make such photo frames important building blocks for AAL scenarios. The results have demonstrated the viability of the concept, but the actual deployment of the system has also shown that the black-box approach with which most photo frames handle cache management may constitute a major obstacle to the selection of appropriate photo frame models. Future work should consider real-world deployment in home settings, allowing additional environmental factors to be accessed and validating the interactive features with other target groups.

References

1. Banks, R., Sellen, A.: Shoebox: mixing storage and display of digital images in the home. In: TEI 2009: Proceedings of the 3rd International Conference on Tangible and Embedded Interaction, pp. 35–40. ACM, New York (2009)
2. Sellen, A., Eardley, R., Izadi, S., Harper, R.: The whereabouts clock: early testing of a situated awareness device. In: CHI 2006: CHI 2006 Extended Abstracts on Human Factors in Computing Systems, pp. 1307–1312. ACM, New York (2006)
3. Consolvo, S., Roessler, P., Shelton, B.E., LaMarca, A., Schilit, B., Bly, S.: Technology for care networks of elders. IEEE Pervasive Computing 3(2), 22–29 (2004)
4. O'Hara, K., Harper, R., Unger, A., Wilkes, J., Sharpe, B., Jansen, M.: Txtboard: from text-to-person to text-to-home. In: CHI 2005: CHI 2005 Extended Abstracts on Human Factors in Computing Systems, pp. 1705–1708. ACM, New York (2005)
5. Sellen, A., Harper, R., Eardley, R., Izadi, S., Regan, T., Taylor, A.S., Wood, K.R.: Homenote: supporting situated messaging in the home. In: CSCW 2006: Proceedings of the 2006 20th Anniversary Conference on Computer Supported Cooperative Work, pp. 383–392. ACM, New York (2006)
6. Burbeck, S.: Applications programming in smalltalk- 80(tm): How to use model-view-controller (mvc)

System Approach to AAL Applications:
A Case Study

Lenka Lhotska[1], Jan Havlik[2], and Petr Panyrek[3]

[1] Department of Cybernetics, Faculty of Electrical Engineering
Czech Technical University in Prague, Technická 2, CZ–16627 Prague 6
[2] Department of Circuit Theory, Faculty of Electrical Engineering
Czech Technical University in Prague, Technická 2, CZ–16627 Prague 6
[3] HIGH TECH PARK, Rašínovo nábřeží 56, CZ–12800 Prague 2
lhotska@fel.cvut.cz, xhavlikj@fel.cvut.cz,
Petr.Panyrek@combitrading.cz

Abstract. The objective of AAL and home care is a better care for frail individuals (elderly chronic and disabled patients) in a home care setting. To improve this kind of care means to allow the citizens to stay at home as long as possible, delaying the institutionalization of people, possibly avoiding it for a high percentage of them. Recent development in ICT shows that it is almost impossible to design and implement an AAL system as fixed to certain hardware, operating system, and infrastructure. Thus it is necessary to develop such architectures that will be easily extensible and modifiable. We will discuss such approaches in the paper.

Keywords: assistive technologies, HomeBrain, health monitoring, ambient assisted living.

1 Introduction

The objective of AAL and home care is a better care for frail individuals (elderly chronic and disabled patients) in a home care setting. To improve this kind of care means to allow the citizens to stay at home as long as possible, delaying the institutionalization of people, possibly avoiding it for a high percentage of them. Institutionalized elderly citizens are at high risk of cognitive impairment, functional loss, social isolation, or death. [6,7]

Integrating information deriving from different sources and implementing it with knowledge discovery techniques allows medical and social actions to be appropriately performed with reliable information, in order to improve quality of life of patients and care–givers. To stay at home means to keep independency, self–sufficiency, social network role.

Currently the mobile technologies, sensors and other devices enable collecting vast amount of data of individuals. This multi–parametric data may include physiological measurements, genetic data, medical images, laboratory examinations and other measurements related to a person's activity, lifestyle and surrounding

J. Bravo, R. Hervás, and V. Villarreal (Eds.): IWAAL 2011, LNCS 6693, pp. 151–158, 2011.
© Springer-Verlag Berlin Heidelberg 2011

environment. There will be increased demand on processing and interpreting such data for accurate alerting and signalling of risks and for supporting healthcare professionals in their decision making, informing family members, and the person himself/herself.

Recent development in ICT shows that it is almost impossible to design and implement an AAL system as fixed to certain hardware, operating system, and infrastructure. Thus it is necessary to develop such architectures that will be easily extensible and modifiable. We will discuss examples of such approach in next sections together with our suggestion of integration of the topic into educational process.

2   Motivation

The main idea is to design and develop an integrated platform (both hardware and software) that would help people especially in their home environment when they are suffering from certain disabilities or have to perform rehabilitation after an injury or brain stroke or "only" help increase their well–being.

Till now most of the solutions are represented by isolated tools, devices or pieces of software. But many of the health problems are rather complex and thus need complex approach to assistance.

For example, a person after a brain stroke has certain motoric problems and also speech problems. It is necessary to perform rehabilitation in both directions and also evaluate results jointly. The rehabilitation process must be monitored as objectively as possible. That means using defined measurement and evaluation of measured data. It is difficult to estimate progress of rehabilitation only from subjective observations. Training of motoric functions can be monitored by cameras, sensors (e.g. accelerators, pressure sensors). From these signals and images we can evaluate motion range, ability to open and close fist, walking, etc. And we can evaluate temporal development. Similarly we can approach the problem with speech. The person can utter sentences and speech recognition system analyses and classifies quality of the utterance. Again we can evaluate temporal development and see whether there is any improvement.

Similar scenarios can be applied to other health problems or disabilities.

The point is to integrate finally all information from partial processes and evaluate the complete state of the person. That can help both the clinicians for focusing their effort and also the patient for finding motivating solution (to intensify activity where the progress is slower). [1,2,3,4]

2.1   General System Design

The system should be realized as a hierarchical distributed system utilizing flexible software platform, as for example multi–agent architecture. Collected data and signals should be stored locally in a data repository; defined part of the data and aggregated information should be send to a clinical data storage (could be part of a hospital information systm, depends on the concrete solution). The

HL7 standards will be followed. In data and signal evaluation advanced methods known from signal processing and data mining fields will be used. It is highly advisable to use defined standard on all levels of data storage, communication, and processing.

One of the key issues is also proper design of sensor network necessary for corresponding data collection. The network should be optimized, i.e. using minimum set for acquisition of maximum relevant data according to the diagnosis and therapy of the concrete person. [8]

2.2   New Technologies Closer to People

The 21st century brings many new technological achievements into our lives. However at the same time there are many challenges connected with high–tech. Quite frequently they appear on the social level – many potential users are not prepared to become the users. Not everybody is technically skilled and not everybody wants to read long and complicated manuals that are sometimes written in a very difficult style (even for technically educated people). Having in mind that the potential users may recruit from senior or handicapped population the user interface must be adapted to their needs.

One of the most significant achievements is definitely the internet, as a break–point in communication platforms. It provides an infrastructure for various technologies that can dramatically improve quality of our lives and make lives more pleasant. Imagine a device that would perform many needed household tasks, monitor our health state and thus become a "home brain" for us. This idea has been behind the project described as an example of integrating platform in the Section 4.

3   Centre of Assistive Technologies Project

We have established a specialized facility - Centre of Assistive Technologies composed of several laboratories and working places: smart home, medical technology and biosignal laboratory, audio/video media laboratory, communication laboratory, and computer/seminar room. The first two are the core of the centre, the remaining three serve for education and research in connected areas and provide also support for the main part. The medical technology and biosignal laboratory has three sections, namely fully equipped intensive care unit (ICU), EEG laboratory (where also other biosignal measuring devices are placed) and medical technology section. This laboratory is focused on research and education that is closely linked with medicine. The intention is to introduce to students most of the technology they can meet in hospitals and in some cases in home environment. They have to understand the processes from the technical point of view. For example, at ICU there is also complete installation of electric power and data networks as in hospitals because the hospital installations have to satisfy more strict requirements concerning electric safety. Here we add new sensors that allow additional monitoring of the patient with respect to his/her safety, state of the bed, etc. The main idea is to design and develop approaches and successively devices that will be able to indicate certain medical problems, one of them indicated by medical doctors is hydration of the patient. Currently only indirect evaluation is done, namely volume of urine. In this area also research connected with electromagnetic compatibility, interference of wireless communication with medical devices will be performed.

The smart home is a test bed for design and development of different setups and functions that can be finally used in inhabited homes. The basic functions currently prepared are: security, control of home appliances, monitoring persons activity, and monitoring persons health state. Now we describe individual functions and technology behind. Security means protection against intruders and we add also safety in the environment. For the security function we can use cameras, PIR-based motion detectors, detectors of open/closed windows and doors. Safety function should control whether specified devices and home equipment are in required state, e.g. whether iron or cooker are switched off when leaving the home, or whether the water tap is closed. Monitoring persons daily activity is important when the person lives alone and has certain disabilities. Then we have to check whether the person is doing well, has not fallen down and injured. Another case is prescribed physical activity or rehabilitation, e.g. after an injury, brain stroke or when multiple sclerosis is diagnosed. Here we can make use of sensors installed for security function and additionally accelerometers, tactile sensors, etc. Monitoring persons health state can make use of the knowledge and skills acquired in the medical technology and biosignal laboratory. Only for personal monitoring we need miniaturized devices. Again according to the diagnosed health state we can propose corresponding setup of measuring equipment (e.g. ECG, blood sugar, blood pressure, body temperature, transpiration, breathing). Recent medical studies have shown that especially in elderly population there is problem with food and liquid intake. So one of the challenges is to monitor unobtrusively and relatively precisely how well the person is nourished. On the

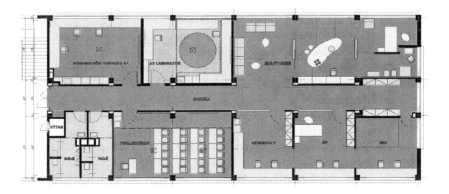

Fig. 1. Ground plan of CAT

other hand at obese people it would be welcome to monitor amount of food and provide recommendation and warning against excessive food intake.

The facility will serve for practical project–based education of students in assistive technologies (AT). The situation in the given field may be characterized in following way: there are no graduates specialized in AT; there is no complex educational program in AT; there exist a number of information barriers between disciplines that may be solved exclusively by consistent interdisciplinary integration; there exists social and objective demand for employees in AT; in the Czech Republic there are relatively many SMEs and institutions focused on AT that need graduates and support for life long learning of current employees. The courses will become a core of an interdisciplinary study branch in Master study and at the same time they will be offered in life long learning. The core courses cover the following topics: data sensing and transmission; sensors, security and control in assistive environment; circuitry and system principles of electronic devices for AT; advanced methods of data mining and knowledge discovery and their applications in AT; telecommunication equipment and systems for AT; multimedia technology. The topics are systematically and logically interconnected. The content is designed in such a way that theory, applications and system integration are represented in suitable proportion.

The Centre will serve as a platform both for education and for applied research in the area of AAL. The main idea is to offer space for development of integrating solutions. Currently there are many partial solutions of smart homes, home security, health state monitoring, internet services. The problem is that these applications have been developed separately and usually they work as closed systems without possibility to interconnect them. The aim is to offer a standard user interface and communication for interconnection of various services and devices.

4   Case Study: HomeBrain – TV Computer

A new project has been started by a Czech company High Tech Park in co-operation with several other companies. The main idea is to integrate many different functions and unify the control interface. Actually the user interface is the core of the project with the aim to have the system control as simple and intuitive as possible. A TV computer serves as the user interface and can be easily controlled in the same way as a standard TV set. The authors have named the project HomeBrain. It fulfils several main functions, namely gate to the internet, multimedia services, senior monitoring, health state monitoring, social networking of HomeBrain users, remote control of home devices, intelligent security system. Additionally, it can be connected to telebanking, e–services (including e–government), and other electronic services. HomeBrain is an example of an integration platform that provides the user with a relatively simple interface. It can be easily extended by newly developed modules. This feature also means that the configuration can be designed on demand based on the user requirements because not everybody wants to have complete set of all possible functions and installed devices. [5,9]

The designers have defined several basic requirements on the HomeBrain. It must be small, having the size of a common TV set–top box and being easily controllable without any need to study a long and complex manual. The Home-Brain device installation is simple – it only needs to be connected to the TV set and internet. Thanks to the new Atom processor (Intel company) the HomeBrain can offer very good technical characteristics. Microsoft environment is used for development of applications and interconnection with other technologies.

Let us focus now on the typical functionalities of the HomeBrain system. In addition to classic TV programs it is possible to watch programs on Internet TV. Search for selected music can be easier – no need to try to find a particular CD or DVD in boxes or stands. Music can be downloaded from the internet (using legal way), or from a storage on the hard disk and stored in the catalogue. Movies can

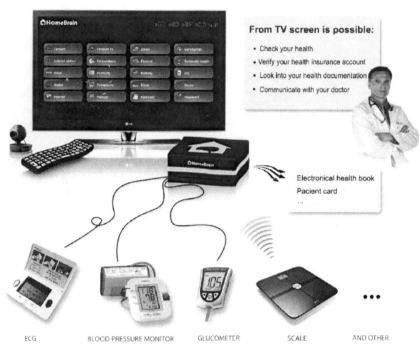

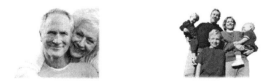

Fig. 2. HomeBrain – TV computer

be lend in a virtual rental store. Browsing digital photographs, creating albums and sharing them with friends is another pre–defined function.

If the user wants to control home appliances remotely on the TV, phone, or via internet the system is easily extensible. The only condition is that the home appliances have the option of remote control. Another possible function is intelligent security. The user interface is interconnected with the installed security system and allows intelligent evaluation.

Eshop is another option. It can be comfortable for elderly people, for people with motoric disabilities or even for ill people. There is a special service that uses bar code reader. Thus regularly bought food can be easily ordered again. The information is sent from the reader to the HomeBrain and then the list of required items is sent to the particular eshop. Of course, necessary condition is existence of such a shop in relatively close distance.

Health state monitoring is becoming more and more important area of AAL applications. Heart–attacks, diabetes, increased cholesterol are typical manifestations of unhealthy lifestyle at present time. Timely anticipation of such state can save lives. Another group is represented by chronically ill persons who must be regularly checked (or even monitored over longer time span). There have been developed many different applications using various sensors and devices for measurement of physiological values. The HomeBrain has an interface for data transfer from such sensors or devices. The user can decide whether the health state information is only stored locally or also sent to his/her family doctor.

The system also offers a similar function to Skype, namely remote contact with other family members or friends living in distant places. There are more functions ready, i.e. calendar, e–mail, video calls, sms messaging, telebanking, e–services (e.g. contact with local authorities), monitoring elderly family members remotely, internet browsing, games. Functions that depend on external services can be active only if the services are available at the given location. This concerns, for example, delivery of food ordered in the eshop, electronic contact to local authorities.

5   Conclusion

We have presented an example of integration platform that allows adding new functional modules in "plug–and–play" manner. An important issue concerns data and its format for storage and communication. Many existing systems are not interoperable because they use proprietary formats and not any existing standard. In such applications as AAL systems that assume gradual extension and adding of new components represents standardization very important requirement. We also believe that it is necessary to introduce all these topics in engineering education. Thus we have designed project– and problem–based education in assistive technologies. A new facility – Centre of Assistive Technologies – has been established. It will serve for students work and application research projects.

Acknowledgement

This work has been supported by the ENIAC JU Project MAS "Nanoelectronics for Mobile Ambient Assisted Living (AAL) Systems" and the research program No. MSM 6840770012 of the Czech Technical University in Prague (sponsored by the Ministry of Education, Youth and Sports of the Czech Republic).

References

1. Celler, B.G., Earnshaw, W., Ilsar, E.D., Betbeder-Matibet, L., Harris, M.F., Clark, R., Hesketh, T., Lovell, N.H.: Remote monitoring of health status of the elderly at home. A multidisciplinary project on aging at the university of new south wales. International Journal of Bio-medical Computing 40(2), 147–155 (1995)
2. Chan, M., Esteve, D., Escriba, C., Campo, E.: A review of smart homes – present state and future challenges. Computer Methods and Programs in Biomedicine 91(1), 55–81 (2008)
3. Costin, H., Rotariu, C., Morancea, O., Andtuseac, G., Cehan, V., Felea, V., Alexa, I., Costin, C.: Complex telemonitoring of patients and elderly people for telemedical and homecare services. In: New Aspects of Biomedical Electronics and Biomedical Informatics, August 20-22, pp. 183–187 (2008)
4. Dang, S., Golden, A.G., Cheung, H.S., Roos, B.A.: Telemedicine Applications in Geriatrics. Brocklehurst's Textbook of Geriatric Medicine and Gerontology, pp. 1064–1069. W.B. Saunders, Philadelphia (2010)
5. HIGH TECH PARK: Project3B HomeBrain (2011), http://www.htpark.eu/en/solutions/r1-project3b-homebrain/
6. John, P.D.S., Montgomery, P.R., Kristjansson, B., McDowell, I.: Cognitive scores, even within the normal range, predict death and institutionalization. Age and Ageing 31(5), 373–378 (2002)
7. Molaschi, M., Scarafiotti, C., Chiantelassa, D., Magnano, A., Ferrario, E.: Evaluation of cognitive and behavioral status of institutionalized elderly. follow-up two and seven years. Archives of Gerontology and Geriatrics 26(1), 335–342 (1998)
8. Rialle, V., Lamy, J.B., Noury, N., Bajolle, L.: Telemonitoring of patients at home: a software agent approach. Computer Methods and Programs in Biomedicine 72(3), 257–268 (2003)
9. Zdravotnické noviny: New project for elderly in Czech republic, thay will have not to be instituonalized (2011) (in Czech), http://www.zdn.cz/clanek/zdravotnicke-noviny/v-cr-se-chysta-projekt-pomoci-seniorum-nebudou-muset-do-ustavu-449873

A Presence-Aware Smart Home System (PASH)

Ernesto Garcia Davis[1] and Anna Calveras Augé[1,2]

[1] Department of Telematic Engineering, Universitat Politècnica de Catalunya
C/Jordi Girona 1-3, Mòdul C3, 08034 Barcelona, Spain
{ernesto.garcia,anna.calveras}@entel.upc.edu
[2] i2CAT Foundation, Barcelona, Spain

Abstract. Wireless Sensor Networks are providing tremendous benefit for a number of industries. A subset of sensed data collected by these networks is presence information. A smart home control system can be designed based on presence information provided by all devices or objects in the home, and we can act depending on it. For this reason, in this paper we present a Presence-aware Smart Home System. We explain its components and features that facilitate the daily living of person's own home.

Keywords: Presence information, embedded devices, wireless sensor networks, ambient assisted living, smart home.

1 Introduction

Wireless Sensor Networks (WSNs) consist of small distributed sensor nodes capable of communicate in a wireless network. WSNs are able to capture a rich set of context information (e.g. spatial, physiological and environmental data). In recent years, the intensive research of WSNs is enabling a broad range of ubiquitous computing applications. These networks are moving beyond mere monitoring of sensed data towards its adoption for environments providing active assistance such as Ambient Assisted Living (AAL) [1]. Also, there is a variation of WSNs that is rapidly attracting interest among research community, namely Wireless Sensor and Actuator Networks (WSANs) [2]. In this case, the devices deployed in the environment are not only able to sense environmental data, but also to react by affecting the environment with their actuators.

A subset of context information captured by sensor nodes can contain information related to user presence. It refers all the determining factors around communication between users or devices (such as their availability, willingness, environment, preferences, etc). Traditionally, only people use this service by means of personal applications such as Instant Messaging (IM). However, presence information [3] can also be used by other type of users such smart objects or devices in order to discover the availability status, conditions and capacity with the purpose to enhance the interaction with each other. In this paper a "smart object or device" refers to anything that has specific functionality and is able to compute and communicate on its own.

Staying well and comfortable, and feeling safe and secure within a person's own home is an important part of life and plays a central role especially in societies that

J. Bravo, R. Hervás, and V. Villarreal (Eds.): IWAAL 2011, LNCS 6693, pp. 159–166, 2011.

have an increasing proportion of older people. One of the objectives of AAL [1] concept is to enable and extend autonomous daily living in a person's own home also when that person reaches an advanced age. In this sense, wireless sensor and actuator nodes embedded in a variety of devices such as electrical devices, windows, chairs, beds or doors, could interact with each other, depending on presence information to perform a specific important action.

For instance, commonly, older people have a more frequent nightly toilet visit than younger people. With pressure sensors that detect when a person is in the bed and movement sensors in the bedroom would be possible switch on the lights to create a safe path of lights in the home. In this way one can better orientate and find the way to the bathroom without risks of falling. That leads to the improvement of the personal safety and security.

Moreover, the presence state of devices can be defined by the interaction with the user (e.g. press on button) or detected by a sensor node embedded on the device (e.g. gas detector). Therefore, that will provide to many older people the feeling of living safely and securely in their own house.

Fig. 1 shows an example of a scenario where the user is supported to live in a more confident, safe and secure way. In this case we assume a smoke sensor has detected a fire event, so the actuator nodes switch off immediately the gas service and the electricity service. It shows how the home environment is able to detect potential risky situations, and perform actions for mitigating the risks.

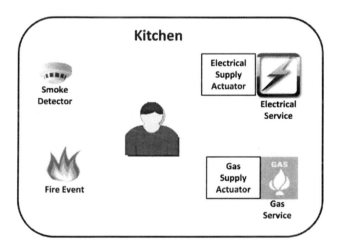

Fig. 1. A general scenario overview with smart devices

In this paper, we refer to our system as *Presence-aware Smart Home* (PASH). It is intended to provide safety, security and comfort at home. Also we explain its main features and components. The rest of the paper is organized as follow. In Section 2, the motivation is described. Next, we describe the components and features of our system. In section 4 we discuss the system functionalities and results. Finally, we present our conclusions and future work in section 5.

2 Problem Description

In the last years, many interesting systems have been developed in the area of WSN for AAL. For example AlarmNet [4] is an assisted-living and residential monitoring network for smart healthcare, CodeBlue [5] is a platform for emergency medical care, SINDI-WSN [6] describes an intelligent home environment for constant monitoring of a patient in a context-aware setting, and Casattenta [7] provides elderly people living alone in their house with adequate and non-intrusive monitoring, aimed at improving their safety and quality of life.

Mostly of assisted living systems are based on centralized intelligence model where a central component is in charge of gathering the required data from WSNs, aggregating data, performing operation and taking decisions to perform an action. Nevertheless, this way of working can generate a bottleneck, due to the increase of traffic towards the central component, leading to network congestion [8] and thus, a low network performance. Therefore, this would result in a delayed taking decision of the system to perform an action.

The features of the network play an important role when we design an AAL system. In the case of WSNs where nodes have constrained resources such as: energy, bandwidth and computing, AAL systems should provide mechanisms to use these resources in an efficient manner.

In most cases, the sensor nodes could report useless data or with a not appropriate data interval to the central component. Generally, these situations are due to the lack of notification mechanisms of the central component to inform about the data the user is interested in and how often it should be received by the central component. Moreover, as various sensor nodes often detect common phenomena, there is likely to be some redundancy in the data communicated to the central component.

In these cases aforementioned, unnecessary packets will be transmitted to the network, thus, it also would result in waste of energy, computing and bandwidth resources on sensor nodes. All of these issues impact the network performance and operation of the assisted living system.

Nonetheless, this model can be improved using a distributed intelligence model where nodes (smart objects or devices) in the system can carry out data processing and taking decisions and respond depending on presence information received. In this way, there is no need to wait for a command from the central component and also it reduces the network traffic towards the central component. Thus it can help to conserve the scarce resources, and reduce the response time of the system.

3 PASH Description

Taking into account issues discussed in previous section, we describe the components and functionalities of the Presence-Aware Smart Home (PASH) system.

These components use the publish/subscribe communication model to exchange presence information. The PASH system is composed of three components as shown in Fig.2.

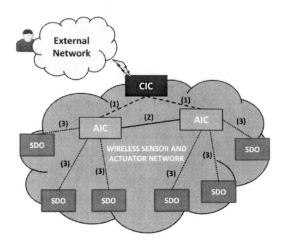

Fig. 2. PASH System Components

1. **Central Intelligent Coordinator (CIC):** It is a central station node (such as PC station). It has at least two network interfaces in order to act as gateway between home area network and external network (Internet). The CIC only exchanges messages with AIC. Fig. 2 depicts this communication with dash lines (1).

   The CIC is responsible of storing the capabilities (temperature, light, window opener, etc) of smart devices or objects (SDO) managed by each AIC, providing administration interface for configuring event/action rules. That means that through this interface the user can relate the event to be detected by sensor nodes and the action that will be performed by the actuator nodes. The CIC distributes this information to the smart devices through the respective AIC.

2. **Area Intelligent Coordinator (AIC):** It is a node installed per section, area or room in the home. It will be always active and connected to household power and used to manage the communication between nodes located in the room, with the CIC and in some cases with others AIC. Fig. 2 also shows the communication between CIC with solid lines (2) and the dash lines (1) depict the communication with SDOs.

   The AIC is in charge of locally storing the capabilities (temperature, light, window opener, etc) provided by the SDOs. This information will be sent to the administration interface of the CIC for configuring the event/action rules as we mentioned previously in the CIC component description. The AIC will act as a broker for the smart devices or objects in its room. That means, it is responsible of storing the status (presence information) of the SDO's capabilities and dispatching it to interested parties (i.e., others SDOs) in its area or in some cases to CIC or others AIC. Besides, the AIC is responsible for data aggregation and reports on demand any information requested for monitoring or administration tasks to the CIC.

3. **Smart devices or objects (SDO):** They are nodes used for detecting events, sensing the environment and performing actions. They are commonly positioned in objects such as windows, doors, chairs, etc. In these cases they are battery-powered

nodes, so efficient energy use is an important issue to consider in these kinds of nodes. On the other hand, there are also nodes embedded on electrical devices, so they use the energy power supplied by it. The SDOs only exchange messages with their corresponding AIC in the area. The circle dotted lines (3) in Fig. 2 depict this situation. SDOs are responsible of registering its capabilities in the AIC, publishing and receiving the interested presence information, and performing a corresponding action.

4 System Discussion

As we aforementioned, the communication between components of the PASH system is based on the publish/subscribe communication paradigm [9] [10]. This is used to publish and receive event information (presence information) of SDOs in order to perform an action for the safety, security and comfort of the people at home.

Unlike traditional publish-subscribe model [9], PASH system is based on distributed publish-subscribe architecture where there are several AIC components located in the different areas, sections or room of the home.

As we mentioned in previous section, each AIC acts as a broker between the SDOs intended to communicate. It means that presence information is only transmitted to AIC responsible in the area. Then, this one processes information and sends to the interested SDO located in the same area. We can see this situation on Fig. 3. For instance, the lights are switched off when nobody is seated in the chair and movement is not detected in the living room. In this case the pressure sensors on the chair (SDO) and movement sensor (SDO), both publish presence information to respective AIC on the living room, and this one processes and transmits it to interested actuator node in the lamp to switch off the lights. This way, the AIC reduces dependencies between interested parties (SDOs), since a SDO interested on event (presence information) do not need to know who is the SDO publishing presence information or the amount of SDOs that publish this information.

On the other hand, the PASH system allows the communication between AICs, in order to exchange presence information between two areas. That means that AIC exchanges messages with other AIC in behalf of any SDO of its area. For instance, (Fig. 3), when a visitor rings the doorbell his/her image is transmitted to the TV that person is watching in the living room. To achieve this objective, the doorbell (SDO) transmits its presence information ("on" or "activated") to its corresponding AIC, this one processes information and transmits it to the respective AIC where the interested SDO (TV) is located. These ways of working allow that only the necessary traffic of data flows through the network, whereas the local traffic is isolated in each area managed by AIC. This is a relevant feature to improve system performance.

PASH system is able to automatically detect new SDOs. That is depicted in Fig 4. When a new SDO enters into the network, it broadcasts a discovery request message (1) to find the AIC in the area. The AIC broadcasts a discovery reply message (2) with information needed for the SDO to establish a connection with the AIC, as shown in Fig. 4. When connection is established between them (3), the SDO automatically registers (4) its capabilities (temperature, light, window opener, etc.) to the AIC in the area. Then, the AIC reports (5) to the CIC for configuration through administration interface.

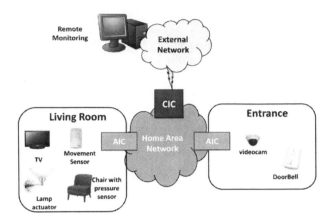

Fig. 3. PASH's general architecture concept

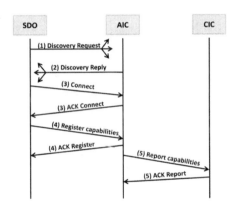

Fig. 4. Example of AIC Discovery, SDO Registration and Report to CIC

PASH system addresses the energy efficiency of the nodes by performing two types of data aggregation [11] depending on the type of component, either AIC or SDOs. In the AIC component, the event publication (presence information) received from SDOs will be aggregated (e.g. by configurable function: average, min, max, status, etc) and will be transmitted in case of data is aggregable. In this case, only one packet will be sent to the interested SDOs. On the other hand, SDOs will not transmit event information to the AIC until a timer expires. They will aggregate in a single message all publication events produced during the timer period and will create only one packet to transmit to the AIC. This technique results in reducing the number of transmissions and thus energy saving of the node. However, there is a tradeoff between the number of transmissions and the delivery delay, since the more the number of gathered data; the less is the number of transmissions. Nevertheless, waiting for more data, it increases the delivery delay resulting in delayed action for the system. This issue is addressed by PASH system, therefore this technique only is applied in situations where network congestion is detected or when an application parameter has been defined by the user.

For monitoring purposes, the PASH system provides a mechanism for querying information in the whole network. This task is carried out through the CIC that is able to query each AIC about the presence information of any SDO in its area. All of this information can be accessed through the administration interface at the CIC. Therefore, this system provides to the user an easy central view of the SDO in the smart home. In addition, authorized users can access the administration interface from external network for remote monitoring, as shown in Fig. 3.

The first evaluations of the PASH system are carried out using the INETMANET Framework [12] of the OMNET++ Simulator [13]. The simulation environment setup consisted of one CIC component and two AIC components with three SDOs each one. Two SDOs from different AIC exchange presence information, the rest of SDOs do the same between the others SDOs through the AIC in the same area. The results showed that the PASH system is suited for providing presence information between smart devices or objects, reducing the traffic flowing in the network around 39%. This shows that the most of the traffic is isolated in each AIC. We are building more scenarios to test the PASH system in different conditions.

5 Conclusions

In this paper, we have presented the PASH system designed for home control in an efficient and easy way. We also show that presence information provided by WSN nodes embedded on devices or objects can be used to perform action to facilitate the home living. That provides older people the feeling of living safely and securely in their own home.

The PASH system addresses the energy efficiency of WSN by providing several mechanisms to reduce the traffic in the entire network through data aggregation. Unlike other projects, the PASH system distributes the intelligence among smart objects or devices and isolates the traffic by room or home area. Moreover the PASH system provides an easy way to configure and manage devices through devices by means a discovery mechanism. The publish/subscribe communication model used by the PASH system allows scalability and flexibility, because of smart objects or devices publishing presence information do not need to know the details of the other devices interested in this information. At the present time, more results are being obtained by simulation. We intend to concentrate our efforts in building and testing a hardware/software prototype.

Acknowledgments. This research has been funded by The Professional Excellence Program IFARHU-SENACYT-Panama and Spanish Government CICYT-TEC2009-11453.

References

1. AAL: The Ambient Assisted Living Joint Programme (2007),
   http://www.aal-europe.eu
2. Akyildiz, I.F., Kasimoglu, I.: Wireless sensor and actor networks: research challenges. Ad Hoc Networks 2, 351–367 (2004)

3. Day, M., et al.: Presence and Instant Messaging Model (RFC2778) (February 2000)
4. Wood, A., Stankovic, J., Virone, G., Selavo, L., He, Z., Cao, Q., Doan, T., Wu, Y., Fang, L., Stoleru, R.: Context-Aware Wireless Sensor Networks for Assisted-Living and Residential Monitoring. IEEE Network 22(4), 26–33 (2008)
5. Lorincz, K., Malan, D.J., Fulford-Jones, T., Nawoj, A., Clavel, A., Shnayder, V., Mainland, G., Welsh, M., Moulton, S.: Sensor Networks for Emergency Response: Challenges and Opportunities. IEEE Pervasive Computing 4(3), 16–23 (2004)
6. Merico, D., Mileo, A., Bisiani, R.: Wireless Sensor Networks Supporting Context-aware Reasoning in Assisted Living. In: Proc. of 1st International Conference on Pervasive Technologies Related to Assistive Environments, Athens, Greece (2008)
7. Farella, E., Falavigna, M., Ricco, B.: Aware and smart environments: The Casattenta project. Microelectronics Journal 41, 697–702 (2010)
8. Chakravarthi, R., Gomathy, C., Sebastian, S.K., Pushparaj, K., Mon, V.B.: A Survey on Congestion Control in Wireless Sensor Networks. International Journal of Computer Science & Communication 1(1), 161–164 (2010)
9. Eugster, P.: The many faces of publish/subscribe. ACM Computing Surveys (June 2003)
10. Tran, D.A., et al.: Publish/Subscribe Techniques for Sensor Networks (May 2009)
11. Abdelzaher, T., et al.: Feedback Control of Data Aggregation in Sensor. In: 43rd IEEE Conference on Decision and Control, pp. 0191–2216 (2004)
12. INETMANET Framework, https://github.com/inetmanet/inetmanet/wiki
13. OMNet++ Simulator, http://www.omnetpp.org

Applying Zheleznogorsk Robotics for Learning Children with Disabilities

Anton Khnykin[1], Nikolay Laletin[2], and Victor Uglev[3]

[1] The Branch of Siberian Federal University in Zheleznogorsk, Russia
antonkhnykin@gmail.com
[2] Scientific-educational Center <<Perspective>>, Russia
laletinnv@gmail.com
[3] The Center for Applied Research of Siberian Federal University, Russia
Uglev-V@yandex.ru

Abstract. The Center for Applied Research of Siberian Federal University and Incubator of Innovative Ideas was set up in Zheleznogorsk. These centers started to operate on the basis of the Branch of the Siberian Federal University in Zheleznogorsk giving unique opportunities for the development of high technologies. The network of educational robotics cluster will link the process of designing robots in a single system; schoolchildren starting to manufacture their first robots will be able to continue their research and design work in colleges and then implement their new developments in the idea of a commercial product. The robotic complex is being constructed to accompany chemistry lessons for children with disabilities (mental retardation, dystaxia, diseases of the musculoskeletal system.). The complexity of the learning process for children with disabilities includes the risk of improper application of chemicals, a needless consumption of the working material and possible danger to health of a student.

Keywords: Applied robotics, chemistry research, educational robotics application, disabilities children.

1 Introduction

Over recent years there has been a rapid growth in developing areas of robotics worldwide, as well as in Russia. This is due to a set up of a large number of affordable items for creating robotic systems and complexes. The company «LEGO™» has made a great contribution to the development of the educational robotics. Thanks to «LEGO™» children all over the world can design robots by using available elements. Currently, many companies are involved in producing robots.

The first World Robot Olympiad was held in 2004 and began an annual forum for schoolchildren competing in both speed and accuracy in making robots. Russia holds a leading position in the educational robotics winning prizes at the World Robot Olympiad. In 2009, two teams became the top five winners of Olympiad on Robotics in

J. Bravo, R. Hervás, and V. Villarreal (Eds.): IWAAL 2011, LNCS 6693, pp. 167–171, 2011.
© Springer-Verlag Berlin Heidelberg 2011

South Korea – a team from St. Petersburg took the third place in the category, and a team from Zheleznogorsk took fourth place in another category. This success was not accidental.

2   Related Works in Zheleznogorsk Robotics

The Branch of Siberian Federal University in Zheleznogorsk contributes to developing of robotics where all schoolchildren involved in robotics are supervised by experienced tutors.

Zheleznogorsk is considered as one of the most technologically advanced cities in Russia where space and nuclear industry is successfully developing. Global navigating system «GLONASS» operated by satellites was created in this city, and the satellite itself according to the author can be considered as a part of the robotic system. In 2008, the Center for Applied Research of Siberian Federal University and Incubator of Innovative Ideas was established in Zheleznogorsk. These centers started to operate on the basis of the Branch of Siberian Federal University in Zheleznogorsk, giving unique opportunities for the development of advanced technologies in Krasnoyarsk Territory.

The partnership of these centers insures a rapid development of the robotics. Several short-term intensive schools for students interested in robotics were held in 2009-2010. Students presented a project «Competition with artificial intelligence» at regional exhibitions last year.

The most significant event of 2009-2010 was the festival of scientific and technological creativity «Robots. Intelligent Space Systems». It brought guests together from different cities of Krasnoyarsk region, as well as guests from St. Petersburg. Competitions were held in different categories and participants of all ages presented their models.

In addition, a network of the educational cluster was established, «Robots. Science and Life». This project gained support from leaders of political, industrial and educational spheres in Krasnoyarsk Territory. This was the beginning of the transformation of Zheleznogorsk into the Robotics Resource Center of Russia.

The Laboratory of robotics is being actively developed – both students and schoolchildren receiving new knowledge in the field of the robotic systems. The experience of the laboratory allows us to develop very ambitious projects.

3   Robotics in Learning Chemistry Lessons for Children with Disabilities

One project we consider in more detail is the robotic complex for learning chemistry.

Chemistry as a science is rather complicated and requires not only the knowledge of theoretical material, but also the ability to apply it in practice, regardless of the physical and mental capabilities of a student. Without independent work with the reagents in the laboratory, any theoretical knowledge loses its relevance.

The robotic complex is being constructed to accompany chemistry lessons for children with disabilities (mental retardation, dystaxia, diseases and defects of the musculoskeletal system, etc.). The complexity of the learning process for children with disabilities includes the risk of improper application of chemicals, a needless consumption of the working material and possible danger to health of a student.

For example, some chemicals can be spilled or improper reagents can be mixed in wrong proportions, therefore there is a possibility of getting chemicals on the skin and mucous membranes of the student's body.

To avoid such effects the robotic system combining the principles of interactivity and individualization of education and safe practical work was designed.

Generally, the structure can be represented as a combination of the following subsystems (Figure 1):

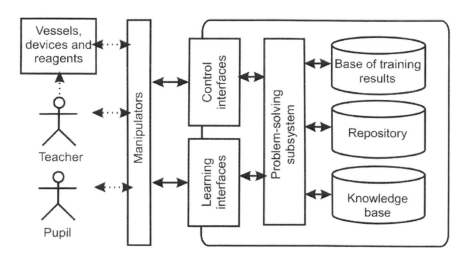

Fig. 1. The scheme of information exchange in the robotic complex

Vessels - (special flasks and test tubes), devices (burners, centrifuges) and reagents - elements of the working environment used for tasks or demonstrations of chemical experiments;

Manipulators - devices for manipulating objects in the environment operated by the students or by the complex (able to block certain direction under the circumstances);

Learning interfaces - mechanisms to dialogue between the user and the complex through demonstration of educational material, its control, the explanation of errors and so on (the teacher prepares all the reagents and vessels beforehand);

- **Control interfaces** - interfaces for configuring the complex and operating the educational objectives (recording, delete);
- **Problem-solving subsystem** - intelligent mechanisms that produce a reaction of the automated training robotic system to the actions of a student or a teacher drawing on the knowledge base, the base of training results and the repository of educational objectives;
- **The base of training results** - keeping the information about users, their marks and individual learning parameters;
- **The knowledge base** - a description of the student' model and the risks of his conduct, as well as automated methods of demonstration of the experiment;
- **The repository** – a file of learning tasks including a demonstration of experiments and the standards of its performance.

In fact, this complex consists of a table (work environment) with operating elements and display, as well as the manipulators driven directly by human hands to perform operations with objects located on the table.

Information system controlling the logic of the robot operates on data coming from the manipulators, as well as diagnoses the learning situation regarding the current state (action) on the table, comparing it with the standards from the repository and with the model of student's behavior.

Complex analysis of a set of training factors is realized through a combination of mechanisms of artificial intelligence (expert systems, semantic networks and frames, fuzzy logic) and advanced educational technology in automation (e-learning courses, instructional testing, cognitive maps of knowledge diagnosis).

As a result, it becomes possible to automate the process of presenting the educational material, the processes of controlling and demonstrating the standard actions, and the process of controlling the students' implementation of practical experiments.

4 Conclusions

New opportunities can be implemented on the basis of previously established Center for Applied Research. We should admit that the need to move educational robotics of Zheleznogorsk to the next level is evident. Using «LEGO™» items is useful for creating simple models of the robotic systems, but more complicated systems require more complex elements; these are all conditions for manufacturing such elements in Zheleznogorsk. Our students can go through the whole cycle of design and construction of the robotic systems at the Centre for Applied Studies.

Functionally, the Center for Applied Research will be a place where students can simulate the robotic system in a special editor. It will automate the assembling process and avoid reworking the robot in the future in case of inconsistency with the task. Afterwards, the simulated robot can be assembled from standard components of «LEGO™» to verify the accuracy of generated models. And finally, it is possible to assemble a complete robotic system that can be put into limited production and sold as a commercial product.

In order to succeed, the project will need to pass the complex path, beginning from renovating and laboratory equipment of the Center for Applied Research, as well as the modern computing system including the facilities to connect to the supercomputer of Siberian Federal University in Krasnoyarsk. However, the intended target disciplines project participants to work together to achieve it.

The network educational robotics cluster will link the process of creating robots in a single system and schoolchildren starting to manufacture their first robots will be able to continue their research and design work in colleges, and then implement their new developments in the idea of a commercial product. They will have an opportunity to work together with the high-tech manufacturing enterprises in Zheleznogorsk or organize their own business in producing robotic products. Obviously this niche is empty now. We should not fail in this segment.

References

1. Khnykin, A.: Laboratory of Robotics and Mechatronics, Center for Applied Research. Intelligence and Science, 103–105 (2010)
2. Lalenin, N., Khnykin, A.: Technology training for high technology enterprises Zheleznogorsk, pp. 133–135 (2010)
3. Sha, L., Gopalakrishnan, S., Liu, X., Wang, Q.: Cyber-Physical Systems: A New Frontier. In: IEEE Intern. Conf. on Sensor Networks, Ubiquitous and Trustworthy Computing, SUTC 2008, June 11-13, pp. 1–9 (2008)
4. Yakubovich, V.A.: Theory of adaptive systems. Soviet Physics Doklady 13, 852–855 (1969); Adaptive Systems with Multistep Goal Conditions. Soviet Physics Doklady 13, 1096–1099
5. Fomin, V.N., Fradkov, A.L., Yakubovich, V.A.: Adaptive Control of Dynamical Plants. Nauka, Moscow (1981)
6. Bondarko, V.A., Yakubovich, V.A.: The Method of Recursive aim Inequalities in Adaptive Control Theory. Int. J. Adaptive Control and Signal Proc. 6, 141–160 (1992)
7. Andrievskii, B.R., Guzenko, P.Y., Fradkov, A.L.: Control of nonlinear vibrations of mechanical systems via the speed gradient method. Autom. Remote Control 57(4), 456–467 (1996)
8. Marshall, J.A., Broucke, M.E., Francis, B.A.: Pursuit formations of unicycles. Automatica 42(1), 3–12 (2006)

Context-Awareness in a Service Oriented e-Health Platform[*]

P. García-Sánchez[1], S. González[2], A. Rivadeneyra[3],
M.P. Palomares[2], and J. González[1]

[1] Dept. of Computer Architecture and Technology, University of Granada
[2] Telefónica I+D
[3] Dept. of Electronic and Computer Technology, University of Granada
pgarcia@atc.ugr.es

Abstract. This work presents a lightweight inference system deployed in a Service Oriented Architecture for e-Health. Modules of an Ambient Assisted Living platform are presented and how to add Context Awareness to this platform is explained. An example of a complete workflow is presented in a real-case scenario.

1   Introduction

One of the most serious problem in actual society is the increase of population aging. Its immediate effect means an increase of people with chronic diseases, discapacity and dependency. In fact, it is expected that in 2050 people among 65-79 will be the third part of the global population, that means, a 44% more than the beginning of this century [1]. Due to combined effect of the increased quality of life and the decrease of natality, this older population creates a economic and social challenge for the future. For this reason, the Information and Communication Technologies is the key to better support these new necessities.

On the other hand, Ubiquitous Computing is a booming area. This concept defines the trend in which ICT are integrated in the environment using every-day objects. The goal of Ubiquitous Computing is the creation of environments with non-intrusive and always available connection. This scenarios are also characterized with the user and devices mobility, several network protocols and dynamic device introduction and removal.

Focusing this paradigm in the e-Health area emerges the *Ambient Assisted Living* [2], a concept which includes methods, theories, systems, devices and services that provide non-intrusive support for daily life and wellness based in the context and situation of people with special needs.

One of the projects that tries to advance in the field of socio-sanitary necessities and Ubiquitous Computing is the AmIVital Project[1], whose objective is to

---

[*] Supported by projects AmIVital (CENIT2007-1010), EvOrq (TIC-3903) and FPU grant AP2009-2942.

[1] http://www.amivital.es/

J. Bravo, R. Hervás, and V. Villarreal (Eds.): IWAAL 2011, LNCS 6693, pp. 172–179, 2011.

develop a new generation of ICT tools and technologies for modelling, design, implementation and device operation of Ambient Intelligence (AmI). In particular, the objective is to develop technologies and tools that allow the implementation of a new generation of applications and services, to support independent life and mobility, monitorization of people with chronic diseases, to help people with special needs, and support for family and caregivers, among other objectives. Nevertheless, the final objective of this project is not the creation of applications to meet this necessities, but the development of a technological platform to the creation and integration of services for different scenarios; services that will be developed and used by several organization and companies, so a collaborative and standard-based development is needed.

This paper explain the design of the Context Awareness Service of AmIVital and its relationship with the rest of the platform. The Context Awareness service is user-oriented in two ways: personal context (manages information about blood pressure, weight, ECG, stress...) and ambient situation (temperature, light, other devices...). This service uses simple rules to generate complex socio-sanitary actuation protocols. Due to the subyacent implementation technology, that will be explained in next sections, it is a portable service, and can even be adapted to embedded devices. The designed architecture for this service, based in different and independent modules, allows the creation of new rules and alarms easily.

The rest of the paper is arranged as follows. First, the state of art, concerning all the relevant technologies and existing architectures, is described in Section 2. Then, Section 3 introduces all the modules in the AmIVital project, and Section 4 describes how to apply Context Awareness to the platform. Section 5 presents an example of an e-health use case within AmIVital, describing all steps in relation with the proposed example. Finally, some concluding remarks and future work are pointed out in Section 6.

2   State of the Art

There exist many works related to context-awareness architectures in e-Health, like [3], whose objective is to create a modular and service-based architecture, but it does not use widely accepted standards. In [4] and [5] the presented platforms use these technologies, but only to integrate different bio-medical devices in a home. Huang et al. [6] proposes an OSGi-based platform that uses inference to dynamically choose among available services in the system.

Related to inference on intelligent platforms, authors in [7] propose a complete Ubiquitous Context-aware Healthcare Service System (UCHS), which provides user's requirements inference and relative services search by semantic inference engine (using NMS). CAMPH [8] is a complete platform based in several physical layers to create several functional domains, using SQL to extract context information, but does not allow to add new functionalities in execution time.

Previous platforms have some drawbacks: there is not well-defined communication with a coordination center using shared datatypes and protocols or they have not any well-defined methodology to add and integrate new services.

Moreover, their inference mechanisms are resource-intensive and could not work in embedded devices or be modified in real-time.

3 Description of AmIVital Platform and Inference Engine

AmIVital architecture is divided in three modules that share datatypes, objects hierarchy and protocols: coordination center, fixed gateway and mobile gateway. Fixed gateway manages the Ambient Intelligence in home, while mobile gateway is responsible of Personal Ambient Intelligence. Finally, Coordination Center integrates both gateways in an extensible way and allows the communication with service providers.

All new developed software elements will be deployed in one of the three different computation nodes. These nodes count with several devices, sensors, actuators and interfaces involved in a direct way on system functions. That is, AmIVital is a logical architecture based in SOA and Ambient Intelligence, and raised using a technological architecture and whose fundamental elements are the services. Figure 1 shows this architecture.

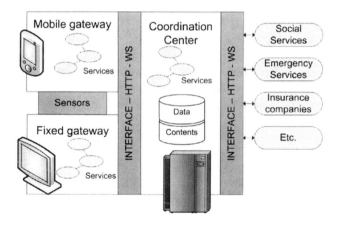

Fig. 1. AmIVital platform scheme. Service providers can add new service to every functional node.

First module, Coordination Center, manages and centralizes user information (medical history, events, multimedia content...) and execute complex business process that involves many project actors (for example alarms, videoconferences, cite management or patient control). On the other hand, Mobile and Fixed gateways manage access to devices that patient uses in his daily life (bio-medical or location sensors, video devices...).

When developing a system like the presented in this work it is necessary to be compatible with the most extended SOA implementations, such *Web Services*. This technology is developed to support machine-to-machine interaction in a network, using several protocols like SOAP, WSDL and UDDI [9].

SOA also can be implemented using other service-based technology, such OSGi. *OSGi (Open Services Gateway Initiative)* [10], is a technology that takes the advantages of SOA to publish and consume services in virtual machines, and provides desirable capabilities to be used in this work, like packet abstraction, life-cycle management, packaging and versioning, allowing the reduction of deployment, maintenance and development of applications. Both technologies are used in AmIVital to integrate its elements.

In order to build the rule engine, the library 3APL-M [11] is used. This is a platform to develop applications through autonomous agents programming, using the 3APL programming language. This tool provides programming constructors to implement facts, goals and basic capabilities (updating facts, external actions and communication actions) of agents and a set of reasoning rules through which goals can be updated or revised. The 3APL program is executed through an interpreter who deliberates on the basis of cognitive attitudes of the agent. 3APL applications are formed by four knowledge mainstays which are executed by the interpreter during executing time. These main structures are described as follows:

- Capabilities: These are mental actions that an agent can perform. The execution of a mental action updates the agent's beliefbase.
- Beliefbase: This contains the information of the agent including its general information about the world as well as specific information about its environment. Beliefs are stored as Prolog clauses (PrologFacts).
- Rulebase: The rulebase contains a list of planning rules; each indicates which plan should be generated to achieve a goal.
- Goalbase: This contains a set of goals separated by a comma. A goal denotes a state that the agent wants to achieve. Goals are represented in first order logic (Prolog).

In our project this rule engine has been configured with a set of rules which allow easily and fast classify the situation of the patient through different parameters. An OSGi package (or *bundle*) containing this service has been deployed in the nodes of AmIVital.

4   Context Manager Service

When developing an AAL Project, one of the targets is to transfer part of the health functionality to the patient's home. To achieve this, it is important to have a complete infrastructure that enables getting all the information of interest about the patient and his/her environment which involves installing a large and varied sensor network.

In the AmIVital Project a lot of different devices have been integrated, like biomedic sensors (pulsioximeters or electrocardiographers), non-biometric personal sensors (activity and location) and ambient sensors (light, humidity, etc.). In addition, the use of questionnaires gives another data source that must be also integrated in the system. After a great work of developing and integration, all this information must be saved in the platform, but if this data is only used to be stored, and consulted from time to time, all this effort does not worth. It is necessary to create an intelligent system used for extracting additional information, detecting which information is more important, examining it and sending alarms if it is needed. In AmIVital two intelligence levels have been planned, so the context awareness is distributed. Figure 2 shows data transactions among systems in AmIVital.

The first level, located in the gateway (fixed and mobile) is executed when a new measure has been obtained or when a new questionnaire has been filled. The system examines each received data to get if an alarm must be launched. At this step of the inference process, only the measures from a single device are evaluated, but multiple measures from the same sensor obtained at different times can be studied in order to determinate if the last one is not within the basal pattern. The inference engine, and the rules over it works, are designed for detecting anomalies and alarms situations, reporting to the coordination center an event with all the relevant information, about the origin of the alarm. In AmIVital, two types of alarms have been considered, warnings and alerts. A warning event only indicates that something remarkable has happened. Otherwise, an alert needs to be immediately attended.

The second step in the inference process is executed in the coordination center. In AmIVital, this second level of intelligence establishes the state of the patient. This level is more complex because of the multiple measures and information sources that must be taken into account at the same time. Data is provided from the gateways or from the questionnaires, or even other patient data stored

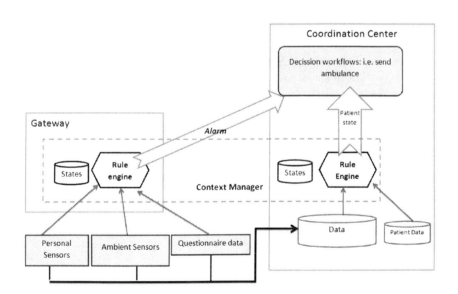

Fig. 2. Data transactions in Context Manager in AmIVital

in the coordination center (like drugs or treatment information). The rule engine works over all this information to obtain how the patient's illness is evolving, checking if the patient's state becomes serious, or if it is stable. As in the first inference step, if there is any change, an event is created with all the relevant information about the cause of that change. Both levels in the context aware-ness use the 3APL application, providing the files that contain the capabilities, beliefbase, rulebase and goalbase structures needed for the inference process. The beliefbase file in particular, contains all the information needed, such as the data obtained by the sensors, information from the questionnaires or even re-sults previously obtained by the rules engine, in order to detect for example, out of the basal pattern values. In AmIVital, in order to try the system, a demon-stration based in a typical disease scene like COPD [12] (Chronic Obstructive Pulmonary Disease) has been developed. The measures available in this scene were heart rate, respiration rate, blood pressure, temperature, pulse oximetry, location, activity, environmental measures (temperature, humidity, etc.) and in-formation obtained from specific COPD questionnaires. When a new measure from a sensor is available, an *endOfMonitorization* event is generated and caught by the context awareness. This is done by the OSGi means. The first step of the inference process analyzes this information using the rules defined for this type of measure and determines if an alarm (warning or alert) must be generated. In this case a new event explaining the cause of the alarm is created. This process is very similar when instead of a measure, a new questionnaire has been filled. For the purpose of the scene defined by AmIVital, the second step of the inference depends on the result of the inference done in the first step. So, only when an alarm event has been generated, this second level of the context awareness is executed, but taking into account all the information available, and not only the one related with the alarm. As an outcome of this, an event indicating a change in the patient's state can be caught in the coordination center. Once an event has been processed a complex workflow is started using the Intalio Business Pro-cess Management System (BPMS) engine[2]. For example, calling to the patient or sending an ambulance to the patient's location. However, this sub-system is out of the scope of this work.

5   Example of a Complete Inference Process

In this section a complete example is described, this will make easy to understand all the process of inference. As it is explained in previous sections, a complete scenario of a patient suffering from COPD has been developed and a several devices have been integrated. The next example is only based in the intelligence related with the body temperature. All the process starts when a new measure of body temperature is obtained from the sensor (in AmIVital, the device used has been the Equivital System[3]). After this new data is available, the *endOf-Monitorization* event is sent and caught by the gateways. At this moment the

---

[2] http://www.intalio.com/bpms/designer
[3] http://www.equivital.co.uk/products/sensors.asp

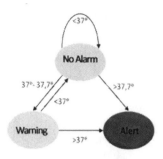

Fig. 3. Intelligence diagram for body temperature measures

part of the context awareness placed in the gateways, takes the measure, and prepares the rules engine, by including the value of temperature in the belief-base. Then, using the 3APL application, and selecting the correct set of rules, the inference process starts. In the case of the body temperature measures, the intelligence developed is the one showed in Figure 3. In this case the intelligence rules can be described using this state diagram, where depending on the value of the measure, a warning or an alert event must be sent. Also past measures must be taken into account, for example, if a *37,3* value is obtained, the result of the inference process should be a warning or an alert event depending of the previous measure.

In the intelligence model proposed by AmIVital, if the result of the inference causes sending an event to the coordination center, the second level of the context awareness is launched. In the case of the temperature, only another source of information (apart from the temperature itself) must be used. In this case, to determine the state of the patient, also information about if the patient is taking antibiotics, is needed. For example, the context awareness service will change the state of the patient from *stable* to *serious*, if the measured value is over 37,7 degrees and if the patient is already taking antibiotics. This change of state starts a workflow in the Intallio engine.

6   Conclusions and Future Work

This work presents an inference service over a service-oriented e-Health platform. The intelligence service behaves as an immediate service (works with only a single measure) or a complex intelligence service engine (obtaining information from several sensors, using different platforms, patient profiles and tests). It also sends alarm events to a Coordination Center to initiate a complex workflow. Furthermore, this intelligent service is rule-based, so it is easy to modify and extend. Moreover, the used inference engine allows the rules and initial attributes to be modified in execution time, so no compilation or system stop is needed. It also has been shown the advantages of Service Oriented Architecture, facilitating the development of all modules by all members of AmIVital project.

Thanks to this advantages, in future work more functionalities will be added, like automatic adaptation or adding new rules to the engine. Also it is planned a more deeper study with real patients in their homes.

References

1. United Nations, Department of Economic and Social Affairs: World Population Prospects: The 2008 Revision Population Database (2008)
2. AAL Association: Ambient assisted living joint programme (2010), http://www.aal-europe.eu/
3. Jara, A.J., Zamora, M.A., Skarmeta, A.F.G.: An Architecture for Ambient Assisted Living and Health Environments. In: Omatu, S., Rocha, M.P., Bravo, J., Fernández, F., Corchado, E., Bustillo, A., Corchado, J.M. (eds.) IWANN 2009. LNCS, vol. 5518, pp. 882–889. Springer, Heidelberg (2009)
4. Pérez, J.A., Álvarez, J.A., Fernández-Montes, A., Ortega, J.A.: Service-Oriented Device Integration for Ubiquitous Ambient Assisted Living Environments. In: Omatu, S., Rocha, M.P., Bravo, J., Fernández, F., Corchado, E., Bustillo, A., Corchado, J.M. (eds.) IWANN 2009. LNCS, vol. 5518, pp. 843–850. Springer, Heidelberg (2009)
5. Baldoni, R., Di Ciccio, C., et al.: An Embedded Middleware Platform for Pervasive and Immersive Environments for-All. In: 2009 6th annual IEEE Communication Society Conference on Sensor, Mesh and Ad Hoc Communications and Networks Workshops, pp. 161–163 (2009)
6. Huang, P., Chien, C., Lee, K., Kuo, Y., Wu, M.: An integration platform for developing context-aware applications based on context reasoning and service automation techniques. In: 11th International Conference on Advanced Communication Technology, ICACT 2009, vol. 3, pp. 1819–1823. IEEE, Los Alamitos (2009)
7. Lo, C.C., Chen, C.H., Cheng, D.Y., Kung, H.Y.: Ubiquitous healthcare service system with context-awareness capability: Design and implementation. Expert Systems with Applications 38(4), 4416–4436 (2011)
8. Pung, H., Gu, T., Xue, W., Palmes, P., Zhu, J., Ng, W., Tang, C., Chung, N.: Context-aware middleware for pervasive elderly homecare. IEEE Journal on Selected Areas in Communications 27(4), 510–524 (2009)
9. Papazoglou, M.P., Van Den Heuvel, W.: Service oriented architectures: Approaches, technologies and research issues. VLDB Journal 16(3), 389–415 (2007)
10. Marples, D., Kriens, P.: The Open Services Gateway Initiative: An introductory overview. IEEE Communications Magazine 39(12), 110–114 (2001)
11. Koch, F., Meyer, J., Dignum, F., Rahwan, I.: Programming deliberative agents for mobile services: The 3APL-M platform. In: Bordini, R.H., Dastani, M.M., Dix, J., El Fallah Seghrouchni, A. (eds.) PROMAS 2005. LNCS (LNAI), vol. 3862, pp. 222–235. Springer, Heidelberg (2006)
12. De Toledo, P., Jiménez, S., Del Pozo, F., Roca, J., Alonso, A., Hernández, C.: Telemedicine Experience for Chronic Care in COPD. IEEE Transactions on Information Technology in Biomedicine 10(3) (2006)

HOMEdotOLD, HOME Services aDvancing the sOcial inTeractiOn of eLDerly People

Konstantinos Perakis[1], Gianna Tsakou[1], Christoforos Kavvadias[2], and Alkis Giannakoulias[2]

[1] SingularLogic, Siniosoglou & Al. Panagouli str., Greece
[2] TELETEL, 14 Kifissias Av., Greece
{euprojects,gtsakou}@singularlogic.eu,
{C.Kavadias,A.Giannakoulias}@teletel.eu

Abstract. Nowadays, the population of the elderly grows absolutely and relatively to the overall population worldwide. Concepts such as quality of life, wellbeing, social interaction and connectivity are of crucial importance, and are directly linked to the home environment. The HOMEdotOLD project aims to provide a TV-based platform with cost-effective services that will be delivered in a highly personalised and intuitive way and will advance the social interaction of elderly people, aiming at improving the quality and joy of their home life, bridging distances and reinforcing social voluntariness and activation, thus preventing isolation and loneliness. The scope of the current paper is to present the aspired personal motivation and social networking services that HOMEdotOLD will deliver to its users, as well the conceptual architecture that will facilitate the provision of these services.

Keywords: AAL, assisted living, elderly, quality of life, personal motivation, social activation, social interaction, social networking.

1 Introduction

Nowadays, the population of the elderly grows absolutely and relatively to the overall population worldwide. Concepts such as quality of life, wellbeing, social interaction and connectivity are of crucial importance, and are directly linked to the home environment, which constitutes the place where elderly spend most of their time for a variety of physical, psychological, psychosocial and cultural reasons. The evolution of ICT has allowed the development of products for the home environment assisting elderly with their daily activities including smart home solutions for devices/appliances management and pro-active remote healthcare. However, social interaction and connectivity support for elderly is lagging behind, given that the main services that are currently available for use by elderly people is standard TV and voice calls. Yet, elderly people, with their accumulated experience and know-how, can become active contributors to society and economy, if given the right means.

Although several social networking platforms, information portals and advanced ICT- means of communication currently exist (both web- and mobile-based), these

J. Bravo, R. Hervás, and V. Villarreal (Eds.): IWAAL 2011, LNCS 6693, pp. 180–186, 2011.
© Springer-Verlag Berlin Heidelberg 2011

applications have been designed mainly for young people and are not so easy to be used by the elderly for the following reasons:

- The average elderly person is not always familiar with technology in general, thus experiencing difficulties in using ICT-based services.
- The user terminals and interfaces provided for such applications are, sometimes, complicated even for ICT-experienced younger users.
- Such applications require experience in complicated registration and installation procedures and maintenance of user accounts.
- New technologies usually impose long training procedures and a high learning curve for the elderly

The HOMEdotOLD project aims to provide a TV-based platform with cost-effective services that will be delivered in a highly personalised and intuitive way and will advance the social interaction of elderly people, aiming at improving the quality and joy of their home life, bridging distances and reinforcing social voluntariness and activation, thus preventing isolation and loneliness. HOMEdotOLD aims at the provision of services through interactive television, as elderly people perceive and interpret a navigation oriented iTV application more effiecntly and effectively than PC-based applications [1]. Even though interactive television has been utilized during the last decade for the provision of services to the citizens, these are mostly focused on the domain of eHealth [2], while communication services even though have been recognized as of significant added-value, they are limited to some commercial approaches of limited functionality [3-6]. On the other hand, the provision of social interaction services has mainly been approached by web 2.0 technologies and are currently provided by PCs rather than TV sets. Social networking websites function like an online community of internet users. A recent survey by AARP, a U.S.-based non-governmental organization and interest group for retired people, has shown that among those who go online, around 37 percent of adults aged above 50 say they use social networking sites like Facebook [7]. In addition, another recent survey highlighted that about one-third of people ages 75 and older live alone, and increasingly they are turning to online social networks like Facebook and MySpace for support and companionship [8]. The scope of the current paper is to present the aspired personal motivation and social networking services that HOMEdotOLD will deliver to its users, as well the conceptual architecture that will facilitate the provision of these services.

2   Methodology and Architecture

HOMEdotOLD will constitute an open platform which will facilitate delivering services that will advance the personal motivation and social interaction of elderly people. Within the context of the project, 2 main categories of services will be developed and delivered to end users, which will also evaluate them during the project lifecycle:

The first main category of services to be provided are the "**Personal motivation services**", i.e. services for staying socially active, preventing loneliness and isolation, enabling voluntariness, motivation and activation. This service category will include services allowing the elderly to perform meaningful activities that are useful and satisfactory for the society and themselves and create new living experiences. This category of services includes:

- a "**social voluntary work**" service, which will run in cooperation and under the supervision of social care organisations, and will notify registered elderly volunteers about several areas of social voluntary work in which they can be involved, thus encouraging elderly people to actively contribute to solving societal problems and to perform meaningful activities that create self-satisfaction.
- "**personalised news headlines**" service, which will provide easy access to news headlines at regional, national, European, worldwide levels, with special emphasis on news that inform the elderly user about the activities of interest (the order and way of presentation of the news headlines will be made in a highly personalised way).

The second main category of services to be provided are the "**Social networking services**": i.e. services for bridging distances and supporting existing roles. This service category will include services allowing elderly living far away from their families and close friends to keep in touch with them and support existing roles. This category of services includes:

- an "**intelligent calendar**" service, which will allow synchronisation of the elderly's agenda with the agendas of friends and family, receiving notifications about possible common activities that can be performed remotely (such as the three types of activities that follow hereafter) or physically, etc.
- a "**videoconference**" service, which will enable –among others– communication with grand children.
- a "**remote dining**" service, which will enable virtual eating together with friends and families.
- a "**photos, videos, experience sharing**" service, which will allow keeping in touch with friends and families and share experiences

Within the context of deliverable D.2.1 of the project, the user requirements were collected and analysed, and the aspired services were preliminarily evaluated by the end users from the pilot sites. The following figure presents the consolidated services and scenario ranking.

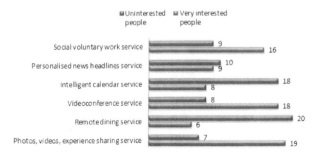

Fig. 1. Services ranking

The users seemed to be especially interested in the "videoconferencing" and the "photos, videos and experience sharing" services, which will enable them to get in touch with their friends and relatives. However, the consortium partners are anticipating the services' evaluations after the users have had the chance to interact with them and use them in their daily life. The services will be evaluated in three pilot sites, utilising two discrete platforms, namely the Philips NetTV platform which will be evaluated by the Dutch and Greek end users, and the AonTV platform which will be evaluated by the Austrian users.

In order to deliver the services aspired, the HOMEdotOLD overall system comprises of five main subsystems, which are:

- The **home environment** equipped with Philips Internet-enabled TVs.
- The **home environment of AonTV customers**.
- The **HOMEdotOLD platform**, where the services logic and data reside.
- The **Philips NetTV platform**, through which the HOMEdotOLD services can be accessed using Philips Internet-enabled TVs.
- The **AonTV platform**, through which the HOMEdotOLD services can be accessed using the AonTV STB and a TVset.

The conceptual architecture of HOMEdotOLD is illustrated in the following figure

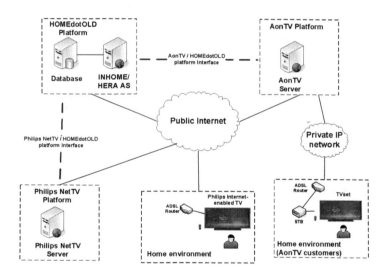

Fig. 2. HOMEdotOLD conceptual architecture

The Application Server architecture comprises of an Apache web server, an open source http server executed both on Linux and Windows, a MySQL Community Server, and the Java Database Driver Connector (JDBC Driver - Connector/J) that enables developers to build database applications in Java.

The main modules constituting the HOMEdotOLD Application Server are:

- The "**Notifications Module**", which is responsible for sending text based notifications to a specific HOMEdotOLD user.

- The "**System Administration Module**", which is responsible for a) handling of creation/removal of user entries in the database and setting of the respective policies, b) maintenance of the news headlines RSS feeds web-sites database, and c) maintenance of social voluntary work openings database (kind of social voluntary work, people required, dates during which the activity is being held).
- The "**Personalization Framework**", which is responsible for providing personalization and intelligence to the HOMEdotOLD services. It includes a) an "**Authentication Module**", which is responsible for authenticating a HOMEdotOLD user, b) a "**Policy Management module**", which is responsible for accessing the database, with the purpose to report to the application logic in which services a specific user has access, and c) the "**Affective modality module**", which user's emotions or other cognitive states and expressions.
- The "**Interfaces with external services**" module, which includes a) the "**RSS Feeds Module**", which is responsible for communicating and extracting information with the news headlines RSS feeds web-sites, b) the "**Picasa Module**", which is responsible for communicating with the photo sharing website, authenticating the HOMEdotOLD user to the Picasa platform and retrieving a list of folders, photos and videos according to well defined configuration parameters, and c) other modules that may be incorporated in the holistic architecture, based on the requirements that will arise during the implementation of the platform
- The "**AonTV Module**", which is the main interface with the Telekom Austria commercial IPTV platform (AonTV) responsible for sending notification requests, and other data, related to the supported services, upon request to AonTV clients.

In this architecture there is an **application logic layer** that hosts the logic needed by the supported services. These are:

- "**Social Voluntary Work Application Logic**", which is responsible for presenting to the HOMEdotOLD user a list of ongoing social voluntary activities and handling user requests to participate to a forthcoming event.
- "**Intelligent Calendar Application Logic**", which is responsible for analyzing the calendar data for all users, according to the data entered both by them and by relatives or friends to the system and send notifications to the users if an activity is triggered. It is also responsible for automatically matching preferences of users and suggesting possible common activities between relatives or friends.
- "**Personalized News Headlines Application Logic**", which is responsible for presenting to the HOMEdotOLD user a list of news headlines, based on the user preferences entered to the system.
- "**Photo, Video and Experience Sharing Application Logic**", which is responsible for communicating with the Picasa module and informing the HOMEdotOLD user when new items are entered in Picasa by relatives or friends. The system presents to the user photo's using a search algorithm

from the Picasa photo sharing website, examining the sharing/viewing attributes of the Picasa folder where the photo has been uploaded. Attributes such as who is allowed to view specific contents is used to present to the HOMEdotOLD user a list of albums and photos.

Finally the **Human Machine Interfaces** (HMIs) provide all the necessary graphical elements so that HOMEdotOLD platform users can access, view, modify their stored profiles and data. These are:

- **"Administration HMIs"** that include a login page and a "HOMEdotOLD Users" page, allowing for creation/removal of HOMEdotOLD users (elderly/friends and relatives) and their respective policies. It also includes a page allowing for administration of the news headlines RSS feeds web-sites and the social voluntary work openings.

- **"User HMIs"** that include a login page, a "Service Overview" page showing the user registered services and a number of application/service specific pages (social voluntary work, intelligent calendar, news headlines, photos sharing etc.).

- **"Friends and Family HMIs"** that include a login page and a number of application/service specific pages (intelligent calendar, photos sharing, etc.).

The HMIs for TV-based applications will be based on the Web4CE framework.

3   Expected Results

The HOMEdotOLD architecture constitutes a pragmatic approach for offering services advancing the social interaction of the elderly. The consortium partners foresee that the development of the HOMEdotOLD platform will facilitate the provision of services that will allow the elderly to stay socially active, will bridge distances and will support the elderly people's existing roles, empowering their social activities.

The HOMEdotOLD platform will be installed and validated in three pilot sites involving real elderly users. The objective of the validation will be two-fold. On the one hand it will enable the validation of the efficiency of the platform and the proposed services as regards their acceptance from the end-users, in order to develop a fully-functional, adaptable and highly acceptable close-to-market prototype. On the other hand, it will facilitate the validation of the acceptance of the platform and the proposed services from a market perspective, evaluating the estimated market intrusion and the possibility for a broader range installation of the envisioned platform.

HOMEdotOLD will enable elderly to live independently with a high quality of life. Older persons shall be able to lead active lives and participate in communities and the society, to socially interact with and even expand their social circle, and to utilize and capitalize on their valuable resources and thus significantly contribute to society. They will be empowered to fight the cascade of deterioration in their health and lives resulting from social exclusion, isolation and loneliness to depression and self-neglect, to maintain and support existing roles as well as define new ones, and to age with their independence preserved.

4 Conclusions

HOMEdotOLD aspires to have an immediate impact on the quality of life of elderly individuals, empowering their social activation and allowing them to bridge distances between them and their social network, thus preventing isolation and loneliness. HOMEdotOLD can play a significant role in the formulation of a more effective and efficient activity-based social activation strategy, which will boost the patients' independence, mobility and quality of life.

Acknowledgement. The HOMEdotOLD consortium comprises of 8 partners, namely the SingularLogic S.A (GR), Telekom Austria (AU), Philips Consumer Lifestyle (NL), Teletel S.A. (GR), Solinet GmbH (GE), Municipality of Kropia (GR), LifeTool gemeinnuetzige GmbH (AU) and National Foundation for the Elderly (NL). HOMEdotOLD will be based on the innovative service platform developed in the context of the INHOME (IST-45061) R&D project, which is already used for the provision of services for people suffering from the Alzheimer Disease in the context of AAL, and on the Philips NET TV platform. HOMEdotOLD is funded under the AAL Joint Programme, call AAL-2009-2.

References

1. Obrist, M., Bernhaupt, R., Beck, E., Tscheligi, M.: Focusing on Elderly: An iTV Usability Evaluation Study with Eye-Tracking. In: Cesar, P., Chorianopoulos, K., Jensen, J.F. (eds.) EuroITV 2007. LNCS, vol. 4471, pp. 66–75. Springer, Heidelberg (2007)
2. Mclaren, P., Mohammedali, A., Riley, A., Gaughran, F.: Integrating interactive television-based psychiatric consultation into an urban community mental health service. J. Telemed. Telecare 5, 100–102 (1999)
3. Abreu, J., Almeida, P., Branco, V.: 2BeOn – Interactive television supporting interpersonal communication. In: Eurographics Workshop on Multimedia, Manchester (September 2001)
4. Quico, C.: Are communication services the killer applications for Interactive TV. In: 1st European Conference on Interactive Television (2003)
5. Brooks, G.: BBC looks to give viewers a chance to chat through iTV. New Media Zero web site, October 24 (2002),
   http://www.newmediazero.com/nma/story.asp?id=237999
6. Pagani, M.: Multimedia and interactive digital TV: managing the opportunities created bydigital convergence, pp. 118–125 (2003)
7. SiliconIndia,
   http://www.siliconindia.com/shownews/About_37_percent_elderly_use_social_networkingsites-nid-68679-cid-sid-.html
8. NY Times, http://newoldage.blogs.nytimes.com/2009/06/01/social-networking-for-seniors/

TALISMAN+: Intelligent System for Follow-Up and Promotion of Personal Autonomy

David Ausín[1], Diego López-de-Ipiña[1], José Bravo[2], Miguel Ángel Valero[3], and Francisco Flórez[4]

[1] Deusto Institute of Technology - DeustoTech, University of Deusto, Avda. Universidades 24, 48007 Bilbao, Spain
[2] MAmI Research Lab - UCLM, Spain
[3] Dep. of Telematic Engineering and Architectures, Universidad Politécnica de Madrid, EUIT Telecomunicación, 28030 Madrid, Spain
[4] Dept. of Computer Technology, University of Alicante, 03080 Alicante, Spain
{david.ausin,dipina}@deusto.es, Jose.Bravo@uclm.es,
mavalero@diatel.upm.es, florez@dtic.ua.es

Abstract. The TALISMAN+ project, financed by the Spanish Ministry of Science and Innovation, aims to research and demonstrate innovative solutions transferable to society which offer services and products based on information and communication technologies in order to promote personal autonomy in prevention and monitoring scenarios. It will solve critical interoperability problems among systems and emerging technologies in a context where heterogeneity brings about accessibility barriers not yet overcome and demanded by the scientific, technological or social-health settings.

Keywords: AAL, health, reactive environment, personal autonomy.

1 Introduction

Accessibility describes the degree to which a device or environment can be used by every person. Nowadays, this term is more and more present in our society, as it is considered a fundamental right as expressed by the UN International Convention about People with Disabilities. On the other hand, technology seems to be present in every aspect of our lives, but it is also moving away from or not giving service to those collectives which most need it.

Effective public access to the benefits of emerging technologies in the Information and Knowledge Society is often limited by the diversity of solutions in both the design phase and in the provision and maintenance of services and applications. National and European policies promoting personal autonomy reflect this fact and, paradoxically, people who might benefit most from ICT are excluded from technological opportunities because of problems of interoperability, accessibility, cost-benefit ratio, security or trust and accessibility in their personal surroundings, such as the home. Consequently, the research pursued in TALISMAN+ aims to provide scientific rigor to technologies that support personal autonomy, laying the foundations of a sustainable, efficient and well thought through development, deriving in the promotion of Spanish industrial activity in this area.

J. Bravo, R. Hervás, and V. Villarreal (Eds.): IWAAL 2011, LNCS 6693, pp. 187–191, 2011.

The rest of this paper is organized as follows: Section 2 summarizes work in technologies related to the promotion of personal autonomy. Section 3 describes the objectives of the TALISMAN+ project and how they will be achieved. In section 4 we define a real scenario in which TALISMAN+ may be applied. Section 5 presents our conclusion and future work.

2   Related Work

Previously created context-aware enabling frameworks and architectures have used different approaches in order to promote personal autonomy. Their analysis allows to highlight the following features [1][2] [3] [4] [5]: a) the context model used, b) the capability of the model for dynamic extension, c) its capability to reason over context, d) the availability of centralized elements, e) resource discovery, f) maintenance of a data log and g) the security of sensitive information captured, processed and stored. From the point of view of reasoning, the first four characteristics are crucial in environmental intelligence settings.

Currently, ontologies are the preferred option to model context in Ambient Intelligence [6] although certain drawbacks have been identified: uncertainty management in modeling of context, distributed reasoning and reasoning for limited resource devices.

Personal autonomy expects that a user working in a ubiquitous computing environment should be able to access both the individual services provided by every device and the complex services resulted from the dynamic combination of basic services. In the latter case, the underlying system should automate or assist the user in such composition process. The different available techniques for service composition [7] require interoperability, for example using ontologies OWSL-S and WSMO.

With regards to security of the information captured, stored and managed in monitoring scenarios, the report [8]from the European Network and Information Security Agency (ENISA) defines a framework to identify the main risks associated to e-health in general and information monitoring and management in particular. Some of these risks do only affect to people individually, whilst others affect to all the users. Currently, apart from the mentioned work by ENISA, there are very few mature initiatives which tackle the mentioned problems integrally.

The applicability of frameworks and architectures for e-health or medicine contexts has aroused great interest among researchers. Indeed, the availability of everyday devices is enabling major advances that are making caring tasks easier in different areas. Mei proposed the development of a framework that would depict patients' vital signs [9] and Tadj, with LATIS Pervasive Framework (LAPERF), provided a basic framework and automatic tools for developing and implementing pervasive computer applications[10]. Roy[11] proposes a framework that supports the merge of efficient context-aware data for health applications that are regarded as an ambiguous context. Finally, and more recently, Preuveneers researched how mobile telephone platform can help individuals to be diagnosed with chronic illnesses like diabetes manage their blood glucose levels without having to resort to any additional system apart from the equipment they presently use, or without having to use additional activity [12].

3 TALISMAN+

TALISMAN+ has four objectives:

1. Analyze and operationally validate in real scenarios the impact and reliability of emerging technologies of multi-modal sensorization in order to generate solutions that are transferable to society to adequately provide services of prevention and follow-up in personal surroundings.
2. Design and implement interoperability scenarios at the semantic level that enable efficient and effective convergence of monitoring and service orchestration technologies that support personal autonomy.
3. Establish mechanisms to define profiles and personal social and health care services based on knowledge that enable agents responsible for running prevention and follow-up services to execute already existing or dynamically composed services depending on the goals or contextual needs, to manage crucial and quality information.
4. Create and evaluate in real scenarios a user-oriented framework for providing services and security guarantees that includes interoperable algorithms and components and enables accessible interaction, either local or remote, of the involved stakeholders.

To achieve them, the project is divided in four subprojects:

— *TALISec+*. It is a framework for knowledge based management of accessible security guarantees for personal autonomy. Its objective is to develop and validate a comprehensive framework that includes interoperable modules and procedures for the provision of e-inclusion and e-health services and applications. It would involve in an accessible and noticeable way knowledge-based guarantees of security and reliability for the electronic management of the information exchanged between actors.

— *TALIS+ENGINE*. It provides cooperative and semantic hybrid reasoning for Service Orchestration in Reactive Environment. The practical effectiveness of undertaking semantic service-oriented modelling of an assistive environment with decision making procedures, undertaken by hybrid and cooperative reasoning engine, in the form of service orchestrations responding to the assistive needs of a user.

— *MoMo*. It proposes a "framework" for multiple vital signs monitoring, noninvasive and accessible. It develops a methodology for defining meta-modules to complement the patient monitoring plan or dependent person according to the profile.

— *Vision@home*. The research aims to develop technology infrastructure and based on vision services for monitoring and recognition of the activity carried out by people at their homes considering ethical questions about the privacy of people who are captured with vision devices.

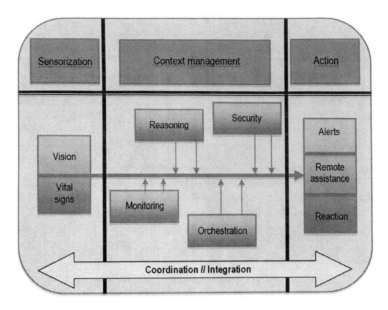

Fig. 1. Logical layers of TALISMAN+

4   TALISMAN+ in Action

Imagine an elderly person with certain level of disability who lives alone and suffers a heart disease. TALISMAN+ may improve his or her quality of life related to healthcare, thanks to:

— *Household activity control.* One of the aims of TALISMAN+ is to get private information about home activity and share it among several devices in order to automatically suggest a response to user's preferences and needs. For example, turning off the water tap when the water level in the bath is higher than a level and there is nobody in the bathroom.

— *Service composition.* In a house, there are several devices which may provide different services. Service composition offers an easy and convenient way to combine them to produce new and more useful aggregated services. For example mixing an external weather forecast with the home's internal temperature and people presence detection to reprogram the air-conditioning system.

— *Health monitoring.* Vital signs monitoring is an important source of information about user's status which allows the system to anticipate a medical emergency such as a heart attack. Anomalous situation detection can give place to the activation of alerting or notification services.

— *Activity recognition.* Vision devices supply information about user activities that can be analyzed to improve context information. An example of an activity that may be recognized and used as context information is sleeping. If a user is sleeping, assisted by TALISMAN+ hybrid reasoning system, media and lighting devices may be automatically switched off or alarm systems triggered in case that the user is sleeping for longer than expected in a non-conventional place at home.

5 Conclusion

TALISMAN+ aims to offer a novel distributed cooperative AAL infrastructure platform offering accessible advances services such activity recognition and health monitoring in order to improve personal autonomy, life quality and care of disabled or/and elderly people. This project financed by the Spanish Ministry of Science and Innovation under grant TIN2010-20510-C04 initiated its work in January 2011 and will implement the objectives and scenario outlined by December 2013.

References

1. Abowd, A.: A conceptual framework and a toolkit for supporting rapid prototyping of context-aware applications
2. Guan, D.W.: Devising a Context Selection-Based Reasoning Engine for Context-Aware Ubiquitous Computing Middleware. In: International Conference on Ubiquitous Intelligence and Computing Hong Kong
3. Baldauf, M., Dustdar, S.: A Survey on Context-Aware Systems. In: Ad Hoc and Ubiquitous Computing, vol. 2
4. Valero, M.A., Vadillo, L.: An implementation framework for smart home telecare services. In: International Conference on Future Generation Communication and Networking
5. López-de-Ipiña, D.A.: Dynamic Discovery and Semantic Reasoning for Nex Generation Intelligent Environments. In: Proceedings of The 4th IET
6. Linnhoff-Popien, T.: A Context Modeling Survey. In: Workshop on Advanced Context Modelling Reasoning and Management (2004)
7. Alamri, A.M.: Classification of the state-of-the-art dynamic web services composition techniques. Int. J. Web and Grid Services
8. European Network and Information Security Agency (ENISA): Identifying emerging and future risks in remote health monitoring and treatment (2009)
9. Mei, H., Wida, I., van Halteren, A., Erfianto, B.: A Flexible Vital Sign Representation Frameywork for Mobile Healthcare. In: Pervasive Health Conference 2006 (2006)
10. Tadj, C.: Context handling in a pervasive computing system framework. In: 3rd International Conference on Mobile Technology, Applications & Systems
11. Roy, N.: A Middleware Framework for Ambiguous Context Mediation in Smart Healthcare Application. In: IEEE International Conference on Wireless and Mobile Computing, Networking and Communications (2007)
12. Preuveneers, D.: Mobile phones assisting with health self-care: a diabetes case study

Stress Telecare Using a Smart Device Controller

Nicolas Boulesteix, Javier Vicente, Begoña García Zapirain, and Amaia Méndez

DeustoTech- Life Unit, DeustoTech Institute of Technology, Univ. Deusto.Bilbao, Spain
{jvicente,mbgarciazapi,amaia.mendez}@deusto.es

Abstract. The aim of this paper is to enable doctors to follow a person's physical state of stress. We introduced a wireless smart device measuring skin conductivity to determine the stress level of a person using the principle of skin conductance. This modification in electrical properties of the skin is related to the activity of the sweat glands. This device can be attached to the body in order to realize continuous measurements. Moreover, it communicates the data using a home wireless network connected to Internet. A battery of tests was performed to verify the behaviour of the system. Two different films with stressing events were used. Therefore, with the help of several guinea pigs, we measured their skin conductance during the entire movies. The times of the stressing moments were the same as the conductance modifications, so we can confirm the correct functioning of the device.

Keywords: ZigBee, Skin conductance, Medical, Domotic, stress.

1 Introduction

Our laboratory has designed a complete home automation system now including a health care system [2-5], located in the patient's house. Thus, the general project is composed of two main parts: the domotic part and the health part. The domotic subsystem will be able to measure several environment data, such as temperature or luminosity, and modify them communicating with the heating system or with the lights. The health subsystem is related to the health of the elderly. The purpose is that of creating smart devices measuring health data directly on the patient's body and being able to send the results to the health service in real time.

In this paper a recently included new part of the project is presented consisting of the creation of a portable stress controller smart device. Stress is a feeling created when we react to particular events. When you perceive a threat, your nervous system responds by releasing a flood of stress hormones, including adrenaline and cortisol. Your heart pounds faster, muscles tighten, blood pressure rises, breath quickens and your senses become sharper. These physical changes increase your strength and stamina, speed up your reaction time, and enhance your focus – preparing you to either fight or flee from the danger at hand. But beyond a certain point, stress stops being helpful and starts causing major damage to your health, your mood, your productivity, your relationships and your quality of life.

We measure stress using skin conductance by evaluating electrodermal activity (EDA). There are two different methods: endosomatic and exosomatic. The

J. Bravo, R. Hervás, and V. Villarreal (Eds.): IWAAL 2011, LNCS 6693, pp. 192–200, 2011.
© Springer-Verlag Berlin Heidelberg 2011

endosomatic method requires the epidermis to be removed and measures the intrinsic body conductance property. The exosomatic technique needs an external current application between two electrodes on the skin.

This wireless smart device is able to communicate with the central command unit [2-5] knowing that this system operates in a ZigBee network. We then created a portable smart device, using the skin conductance method, one that is able to communicate the data thanks to the ZigBee Health Care profile. It detects the patient stress level continuously, without disturbing him, and sends it to doctors in real time.

2 Methodology

2.1 The Communication Protocol: ZigBee

ZigBee [1] is an open global standard providing wireless networking based on the IEEE 802.15.4 standard and taking full advantage of a powerful physical radio that this standard specifies. ZigBee is the result of collaborative efforts of companies known as the ZigBee Alliance. ZigBee includes the following key features:

Table 1. ZigBee Features

Reliability and self-healing	Very long battery life	Ability to be used globally
Support for a large number of nodes	Security	Product interoperability
Fast, easy deployment	Low cost	Vendor independence

ZigBee is well suited for a wide range of building automation, industrial, medical and residential control and monitoring applications. Examples include the following: *Lighting controls, Automatic Meter Reading, Wireless smoke and CO detectors, HVAC control, Heating control, motion or glass break detectors, standing water or loud sound detectors…etc*

Reliable data delivery is critical to ZigBee applications. The underlying 802.15.4 standard provides strong reliability through several mechanisms at multiple layers. It uses 27 channels in three separate frequency bands. The basic 802.15.4 node is very efficient in terms of battery performance. The standard specifies transmitter output power at a nominal −3 dBm (0.5 mW), with the upper limit controlled by the regulatory agencies.

2.2 Stress

Today, stress levels cannot be measured with accuracy. Some methods have been created in order to show a human being's approximate state of stress. The first one, the Holmes and Rahe Stress Scale, consists of listing the modifications in life that a person underwent in the previous 24 months. For this test the patient has to check the boxes in front of the "Life changes Units" in the scale, and then he adds the number of times he has experienced it in the last year. To finish, he adds the different values associated with the facts and obtains a score between 0 and +300.

The score interpretation gives him an overview of his state of stress:

> **Score of 300+**: *At risk of illness.*
> **Score of 150-299+**: *Risk of illness is moderate (reduced by 30% from the above risk).*
> **Score 150-**: *Only has a slight risk of illness.*

The other way to discover the state of stress in a person consists of measuring changes in temperature, blood pressure or galvanic skin response.

When a person is subjected to high stress levels his physical temperature increases, especially in the extremities of the body. However, skin temperature can also increase due to another illness, so this is used in addition to other methods.

Blood pressure is also a biological value changing with stress levels. Like body temperature, it can be measured and translated as a stress value. When a person is under stress the heart works harder, so it sends more blood and the pressure in vessels increases; this is easy to detect.

If Electro Dermal Activity is used as the dependent variable, then skin conductance is usually the appropriate method. The GSR consists of applying a direct current constant voltage probe signal to the skin. Skin conductance is usually measured in "microSiemens" or "micromho" units.

3 Design

Figure 1 presents the general block diagram of the system, and then some detailed diagrams will be added to explain the system more deeply.

Block 1: Power supply subsystem
We observed that we have to put electrodes on the skin of the patient; this constitutes the input impedance of the system.

Block 2: Signal Processing
This block transforms and prepares the signal to be sent keeping the original message, of course.

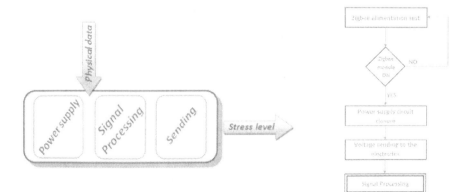

Fig. 1. High level design block detailed   **Fig. 2.** Power supply process

Block 3: Sending Block

Finally, the product's last process that of the sending method. In fact, the integration of the device in a Zigbee network is included in the principal objective of this project.

However, due to the fact that the electrical resistance cannot be measured in direct form, we will measure it indirectly using the principle of V=RI. Thus, we will apply a constant voltage (V) to the patient; with the variation of his skin resistance (Rs), it will produce an inverse variation of the current (I). Afterwards, we can make this variable current pass through a constant resistance (Rc) and we will obtain a final voltage (Vo) corresponding to the patient's skin resistance.

Here you can see the principle in equation:

$V=Rs*I$	*(1)*	$Vo=Rc*I$	*(3)*
$I=V/Rs$	*(2)*	$Vo=V*Rc/Rs$	*(4)*

With: V=applied voltage, Rs=skin resistance, I=current, Vo=final voltage, Rc=constant resistance.

Within exosomatic recording, the applied current can either be direct current or alternative current; and within direct current measurements, the recording can be made with either a constant voltage source or a constant current source.

The simplified representation of the final system is shown in Figure 3. The 3 different blocks of the system can be discerned.

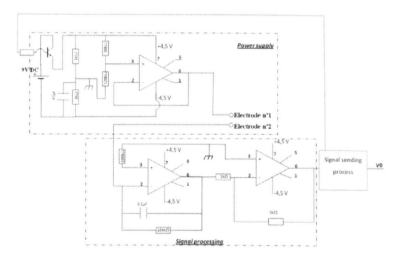

Fig. 3. General diagram including part of the circuits

There are no direct advantages to choosing either method; consequently, measurements will be acquired with the most prevalent method in the field: direct current, constant voltage.

Figure 2 shows how the power supply process operates. So that, it can be seen that the circuit is activated only with the Zigbee module. Thanks to the latter, power waste is minimized and autonomy is increased.

We used two electrodes arranged on patient's skin surface in such way that the skin represents the input impedance of the circuit. The power supply of the amplifiers has to be positive and negative. We created a voltage divider with a new earth point. Thanks to this, we obtain +4,5V DC and -4,5V DC sources. See figure 10.

We decided to produce a second voltage divider to create the needed voltage. Therefore, using two resistances, we created a 3.3 V voltage supplying the measure circuit.

In order to reduce energy waste, we decided to turn off the device whenever the measure was not needed. Indeed, the central network will turn on the ZigBee module for five seconds every two minutes in order to communicate the data. This is why we do not need to realize measures all the time, only during the activation of the sending process.

Consequently, we decided to control the measure circuit's power supply with the ZigBee module, which is why we included a transistor to enable the current to pass through or not.

At the exit of the skin electrodes, we obtain a current varying with skin resistance. In order to increase the voltage obtained after the electrodes, we decided to put in another amplifier. This one will be arranged as an inverting amplifier; with a gain proportional to the subject's skin resistance.

Nevertheless, the voltage will be inversed after this amplifier, so we considered also applying a third amplifier in the inverting configuration, but with a fixed gain.

Thanks to this method, we will obtain a Vo voltage that is clearly visible and proportional to the skin resistance of the patient.

Figure 4 provides the organigram of the signal processing block. Two amplifiers can be discerned: the first one on the left, used as an inverting amplifier with a variable gain (G), explained as:

$$G=Vo/V=-Rc/Rs; \qquad Vo=-V*Rc/Rs \qquad (5)$$

With: G=gain, Vo=final voltage, V=applied voltage, Rc=constant resistance, Rs=skin resistance

Therefore, if the skin resistance (Rs) changes, the final voltage (Vo) will change proportionally. After several tests we decided that the best value of Rc is: $Rc=100k\Omega$.

So, with V=3V, we have: $G=Vo/3=-100/Rs$, $Vo=-3*100*10^3/Rs$

As can be appreciated, the final voltage will be inversed. As previously mentioned, the chosen technology is the ZigBee PRO communication protocol. Therefore, we decided to use a controller based on this protocol to send our data to the central unit. The chosen chip is built by Jennic Company. It is an ultra-low power, low-cost wireless microcontroller for wireless sensor networking applications based on the IEEE802.15.4 standard, including ZigBee PRO and JenNet. The integrated power management on the JN5148 efficiently controls the system power, enabling it to support applications that require the use of a coin cell with a 20mA limited discharge capability. With a system-operating current consumption of 18mA when receiving and 15mA when transmitting at +3dBm, the JN5148 typically consumes 35% less power than existing solutions in these modes of operation.

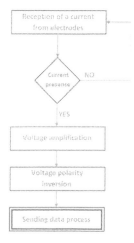

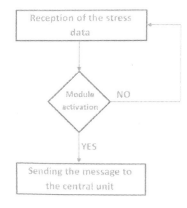

Fig. 4. Signal processing process

Fig. 5. Sending method process

We reduced the main board to obtain a 5cm long system. The entire prototype with all the modifications can be seen in the following pictures. The picture in Figure 6 is a detailed view of the boards, Figure 7 shows the prototype when the two boards are plugged and Figure 8 shows the final electrode design: (using ECG electrodes).

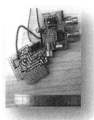
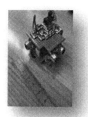
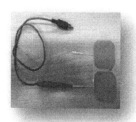

Fig. 6. Third prototype details   **Fig. 7.** Integrated prototype overview   **Fig. 8.** Final electrodes

The box integrating the system and the final shape of the device can be seen in Figures 9 and 10. It should be pointed out that this box measures less than 10cm and contains the circuit and the power source.

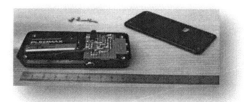
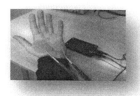

Fig. 9. Open final product picture

Fig. 10. Final product picture

4 Results

All the validation tests were performed with the same recording tool: the PicoScope from Picotech Company. In order to visualize the received signal, we used a computer working with "PicoScope 6" software from Picotech Company.

Concerning the stressing elements, two types of videos were used. The first one is a short video track which is intended to surprise the guinea pig. On the contrary, the second one is a frightening movie, which will enable us to link stress evolution to the movie sequences.

Here is the description of both videos used for the test battery:

✓ The short video is: *a surprising and horror video found on Youtube.com.*

✓ The movie is: ***Tesis,*** *directed by Alejandro Amenábar in 1996.*

The short video test was carried out first because it is the one used for all prototype tests. We therefore knew that the device was actually working with this one and had no doubts in the results. The stressing moment began 40 seconds after the beginning of the test. The first test was performed with Hugo. The reference value of the stress was 0.0144 V.

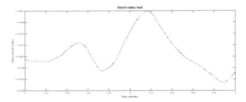

Fig. 11. Short video: Hugo's result

In this test we can observe a 2-second delay in the response. The amplitude maximum (from the reference) was 2,1 mV.

The second test was used on Iñigo (Fig. 12), with a reference value of 0,0175V. The last test was performed on myself (Fig. 13), and the reference value was 0.022V. In this test, the delay is more important, about 4.5 seconds. The amplitude maximum (from the reference) was 5 mV. Here, the amplitude maximum (from the reference) noticed was: 1 mV.

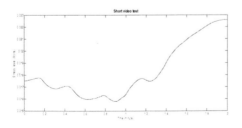 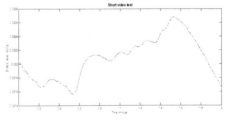

Fig. 12. Short video Iñigo's result   **Fig. 13.** Short video Nicolas's result

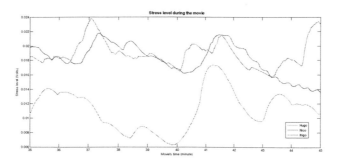

Fig. 14. Results of the three movie tests

Firstly it can be observed that the last test is not very relevant because the increase signal began just before the stressing event. We think that this was caused by knowing about the short video before the test.

So, from the first two tests' results we can say that this device can show skin conductance variation during short stressing events. Indeed, we can appreciate an increase in the signal after the stressing event more or less precisely.

The "Tesis" movie test was carried out on three 23-year-old men. Hence, we have arranged the device on the hand skin of three guinea pigs during the entire movie to show the stress reaction during the stressing moments. Results have been recorded and a comparison made of the ten minutes between 35 and 45 minutes.

Indeed, we can particularly notice an increase in skin conductivity in the 40th minute (proportional to the amplitude of the signal Vo). This corresponds to a previously marked stressing moment of the movie. This fact is visible for the three guinea pigs. so we can say that the test is conclusive.

5   Conclusions

The principal aims of this work were the study and realization of a wireless device allowing measurement of a person's level of stress. This project was integrated into a larger one consisting of producing a domotic health-care system.

This objective thus encouraged us to carry out much research into two principal topics: wireless communication protocols and stress in general.

The most important conclusion of the paper is that the physical consequences of stress can be measured with the study of skin conductance variations. The final design is constituted by a power source supplying a signal processing circuit measuring skin conductivity and transmitting it via a communication port.

The realization of several tests demonstrates that the created device was able to detect the variation of stress. However, the obtained signal has to be compared with a reference stress value. That is why we can consider future improvement of this device by creating a stress scale providing different values of patient stress.

The creation of this smart device enabled us to imagine the new offered possibilities. For example, another smart device which is able to measure different health parameters under a health supervisor device, integrated into a home network, communicating directly with the doctors involved.

Acknowledgments. This work was partially supported by the Basque Country Department of Education, Universities and Research.

References

1. http://www.zigbee.org/
2. Masella, C., Zanaboni, P., Di Stasi, F., Gilardi, S., Ponzi, P., Valsecchi, S.: Assessment of a remote monitoring system for implantable cardioverter defibrillators. J. Telemed. Telecare 14, 290–294 (2008)
3. Hooper, G.S., Yellowlees, P., Marwick, T.H., Currie, P.J., Bidstrup, B.P.: Telehealth and the diagnosis and management of cardiac disease. J. Telemed. Telecare 7, 249–256 (2001)
4. Barlow, J., Singh, D., Bayer, S., Curry, R.: A systematic review of the benefits of home telecare for frailelderly people and those with long-term conditions. J. Telemed. Telecare 13, 172–179 (2007)
5. Scalvini, S., Mazzù, M., Giordano, A., Zanelli, E., Piemontese, C., Fedele, F., Glisenti, F.: A review of seven years' telecardiology experience. J. Telemed. Telecare 13, 50–52 (2007)

Image Processing Algorithms for AAL Services

Iván Ovejero, Elena Romero, Zorana Bankovic, Pedro Malagón, and Alvaro Araujo

Electronic Engineering Department, Universidad Politécnica de Madrid
Avda/ Complutense 30,
28040 Madrid, Spain
{iovejero,elena,zorana,malagon,araujo}@die.upm.es

Abstract. The image processing techniques are widely used in many fields, such as security and home automation. With these techniques algorithms are developed for its use in common vision systems (with regular video cameras connected to a computer), consuming too many resources.

This paper presents some innovative algorithms to be included in autonomous vision systems. These vision systems, included in a Wireless Personal Area Network, allow the development of AAL services, which are able to operate autonomously and in a totally transparent way to the users, making their everyday tasks easier.

1 Introduction

The ageing of the population has produced an increase in personal care needs. New technology developments could be a potential answer to the requirements of a society demanding for better assistance [1]. One of the latest innovations in the area is the Ambient Intelligence (AmI) [2] and AAL.

These AAL solutions often are based in environments which control many features in the home in an automated way. One of the most important characteristics in these environments is that devices should communicate with each other.

Some features are crucial in AAL scenarios. The system must be able to meet our needs with low resource consumption, to be cost affordable and to increase batteries life.

In order to provide extra-features to AAL scenarios, the use of image based sensor could be one of the most important improvements since it provides us enriched information. This information allows us to know in real time, what happens in a room, analyzing the situation and acting for itself. To make this possible, the fundamental step is the development of image processing algorithms able to equip our system with low resource consumption functions, which permit it to detect movement, activity parameters (such as speed and direction of the mobile objects) or inactivity periods (i.e. a fall or a sleeping person). These extra-features will allow us, for example, tracking people with Alzheimer or detecting a fall.

Thanks to image sensor, new services developed could contribute to increase independence of people with disabilities, reduce the risk of accidents, allow quick intervention in case of emergency, and monitor the user status and its house, providing information about his habits, in a totally transparent way for the user, and allowing its implementation in a low-cost architecture.

J. Bravo, R. Hervás, and V. Villarreal (Eds.): IWAAL 2011, LNCS 6693, pp. 201–208, 2011.
© Springer-Verlag Berlin Heidelberg 2011

This paper presents a work in progress which shows some innovative image processing algorithms for autonomous vision sensors, included in a WPAN architecture [3], which will allow the implementation of AAL services, improving the user quality of life.

In section 2, we will review the related works which this paper is based on. The architecture and the services we can provide are described in sections 3 and 4 respectively. Finally, we describe the proposed algorithms, a key part of the system, and the used vision system, analyzing the conclusions derived from the work.

2 Related Work

The image processing covers an enormous variety of possibilities; for example can be used for the implementation of a gestural interface or to develop a mobile robot. In recent years, the development of image processing algorithms in the field of care services has come a long way, helping to improve AAL services. Paper [4] describes tracking people and movement detection algorithms. These algorithms are closely related with the present paper, but are implemented for systems with simple cameras, which resources that the autonomous vision systems do not possess.

In [5] the authors develop a vision application which can be valid for our purpose. They present us an edge detection algorithm for a moving detection implements on a mobile robot. But this kind of moving detection algorithm do not working properly in environments with large numbers of objects, such as houses, laboratories or rooms, due to mixing between different objects' edges.

For AAL purpose, it is important to develop algorithms that can be used in complex environments. In this way [6] shows a frame to frame algorithm for moving detection with an absolute threshold process for bio-microfluidics that could serve as a model. This algorithm solves the above problems, but cannot detect inactivity periods (periods without movement), because the frame to frame analysis eliminates the detection of static areas, hindering the detection of inactivity periods (i.e., sleeping person, a fall, etc...), basics in AAL services.

As noted, we cannot find a common method in image processing that cover the necessities in AAL. In [7] we find a summary of image processing techniques that can be adapted to develop appropriated AAL services.

3 Architecture

The vision sensor has to been included in the AAL architecture, in this case, a WPAN constituted by several nodes (light regulator, vision sensor, etc). Each node has three different parts. First the sensor itself (presence, pressure, vision, light...); second an autonomous power supply; and third the intelligence module, which provides all the necessary intelligence (routing, reconfiguration, process information...). The commonly used OSI architecture has been discarded in favour of a service-based architecture. The aim of this design is to implement applications that arise as a mere aggregation of services and relations between services, rather than a node-focused orientation, simplifying the development of user applications.

In this way, the vision sensor provides enriched information to the system. This information, coupled with the rest of data collected by other sensors in the network will be analysed and processed, allowing the development of AAL services described below. These services are above the architecture, completely transparent for the user, eliminating any human-machine interaction and improving their quality of life [8].

4 Services

As mentioned above, services are built on top of an APP layer that abstracts network or hardware specific tasks to the application. This allows easily compose applications (by the mere services addition) to take into account many complex aspects, such as privacy or safety, in a totally transparent way to the user.

The autonomous vision system provides us enriched information, allowing implementing a large range of applications.

According to the context of this paper, the most appropriated AAL services are described below.

4.1 User Modelling Service (UMS)

This kind of services uses and manages the data to recognize interests, habits, behaviours and needs of the user in a concrete spatio-temporal situation. This information (named context in AmI), which can be obtained by simple processes such as user tracking process and inactivity periods detection process, is stored in a data base specifically designed to this kind of services as an attributed-value pair constituted user profiles. During the execution time, this information is processed and updated, improving knowledge and understanding of user's habits.

These characteristics allow providing specific and personalized services according to the user needs [9], depending on several factors such as week day, season, presence of third person, etc. Thus, the system is completely integrated in the life of the user in a transparent way, making easy the daily tasks and taking care of the health in a non-pervasive mode.

4.2 User Tracking Service (UTS)

User tracking systems are currently widely used in the implementation of security platforms and application for elderly people. This kind of systems allows basic movement patterns identification and future action prediction. These features can be implemented with our vision system, described below. The utilization of this kind of device offers a wide range of possibilities for the above scenario since it is able to detect intrusions, to improve the performance of easy daily task or to identify alarms produced by fallen or by longer user inactivity period.

4.3 Object Tracking Service (OTS)

As well as the service described above, this service could be based on the features provided by our vision sensor, specifically in objects tracking algorithms and inactivity-period-detection methods.

This kind of services will allow us to develop interesting application for the Ambient Assistance field, especially in security issues. One use of these services may be a stolen/abandoned-object- detection application, which activates an alarm when adverse events are detected (i.e. detection of stolen objects or obstacles that reduce the mobility of persons with disabilities).

5   Image Processing Sensor

The main purpose of this paper is the development of algorithms that can be implemented in autonomous vision system. This system must be able to meet our needs with low resource consumption, so the system Eye-RIS developed by AnaFocus is the most appropriate for this purpose. Reasons for this choice have been based on a study of possible autonomous vision sensors available on the market, whose main features are perfectly suited to our needs described below.

This sensor is a vision system that are conceived to be implemented as low-cost and very compact platforms capable to solve complex vision tasks at very high speed and with very low power consumption. It has capabilities in image processing and incorporates enough computing power to perform functions that allow developing applications [10].

The most relevant features of our vision system are:

- Large operational flexibility. Can reconfigure and parameterize the hips to meet the needs of consumers.
- General-purpose, all-in-one architecture including processors, memories, etc.
- Huge computational power with low-power consumption.
- Truly mixed-signal architecture, providing us two process levels. First, the analog input images are processed, eliminating redundant information, and allowing its digitization in order to extract its main features in the later stage, speeding up de image processing.

These features allow developing algorithms which can improve the base of our AAL systems. These algorithms are described below.

6   Algorithms

Up to now, we have implemented two algorithms: tracking people-objects algorithm, and stolen-abandoned object detection algorithm, which can be easily developed, becoming a really interesting tool for our purposes. Both algorithms have the same basic structure describes below:

6.1   Segmentation

The background/foreground segmentation is a fundamental part of any image processing algorithm, allowing differentiating between the constant area (background) and the static and dynamic areas (foreground) that appear in the image.

The background initialization is a crucial part of the segmentation process because should not include any moving or stationary object to be analyzed. Due to memory limitations of the vision system, segmentation methods based on multi-modal backgrounds, such as Mixing of Gaussian (MoG) or Hidden Markov Models (HMM), have been ruled out. Furthermore, frame to frame segmentation methods (continuous subtraction images) cannot be used because does not allow analysing the static areas outside the background. The use of algorithms based on edge detection has discarded too due to the large amount of accumulated objects in the images.

As a result, take a single background image, which may be updated periodically during inactivity periods (periods without movement or static objects) will be the best option. The segmentation process consists basically in the subtraction of the background and the image flow taken at real time, after low pass filtering to eliminate the acquisition noise.

We use a linear Gaussian filter whose template is shown in Figure 1. The pixels of the new image are obtained by weighting each pixel of the previous image with the template.

$$T = 1/16 \times \begin{bmatrix} 1 & 2 & 1 \\ 2 & 4 & 2 \\ 1 & 2 & 1 \end{bmatrix}$$

Fig. 1. Template applied within Gaussian Filter

6.2 Threshold

Threshold process allows converting the image from the segmentation process in a binary image, eliminating redundant information and obtaining its basic characteristics (number of objects, coordinates of mass center …). This step provides relevant information to obtain in later processes more complex features such as speed and trajectory of moving objects. Thus, the images could be processed more easily and quickly.

For the full objects definition, two threshold limits have been defined, obtaining an absolute threshold process. We use the classic expression of threshold process. (Figure 2).

$$Destination\_Image(i, j) = \begin{cases} Black\ (0) & if\ Source\_Image(i, j) \leq Threshold \\ White\ (255) & i.o.c. \end{cases}$$

Fig. 2. Threshold expression

6.3 Processing

This process begins with an erosion/dilation process to remove the isolated points produced by illumination changes and define more precisely the separation between nearby objects. Finally, we obtain the objects mass centre and its coordinates.

At this point, the algorithms begin to diverge:

6.3.1 Tracking People-Objects Algorithm

The algorithm can obtain object speed and trajectory calculating the time between frames and comparing the current and latest coordinates of mass centres. It could be possible that some object parts have the same gray intensity of the background. This result in an object defined by several mass centres that the algorithm grouped to obtain the real mass centre. Identified the object by a single point, next step is apply the previous tracking method.

Another problem occurs when two objects intersect each other. In this case, the system detects a single object (like a "single mass"). To avoid this problem, the system assumes constant object movements and updates its positions in relation to its speed and trajectory. Figure 3 shows an example of the algorithm.

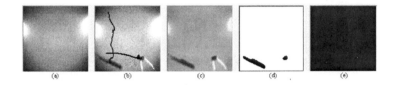

Fig. 3. (a) Background; (b) Image Flow; (c) Segmented Image; (d) Threshold; (e) Mass Centres

6.3.2 Stolen-Abandoned Object Detection Algorithm

The algorithm detects when an object disappears from background (possible stolen object), or appears in the image (possible abandoned object), and initializes a counter. The counter is only updated if the area remains static. If the counter reaches its limit (may vary depending on user needs), next step is to discriminate between stolen and abandoned object. Unlike the existing algorithms that consider image sequences before and after the moment of the alarm, we use a method based on intensities comparison. A disappeared object from the background (stolen object) results in a static area with a low gray intensity, whereas if the object has appeared in the image (abandoned object), this area has high grey intensity. It must take into account the intensity of the background used because it modifies the intensities of the segmented image, producing errors. Figure 4 shows an execution example. In the first image we detect a stolen object, and in the second one an abandoned object. Object positions are marked in both cases.

Described algorithms are the basic algorithms of the services proposed above. With them it can be implemented all the functionalities required based in the information provided by them (inactivity periods, moving objects and its trajectories, etc). These implementations work with low resources consumption and in a fast and simple way. These algorithms can be useful too in other areas, such as security application for stolen object detection, following the thief movements, or industrial control application that allow detecting falling objects or structural damage (cracks, leaks…), forming a powerful tool for the development of autonomous systems.

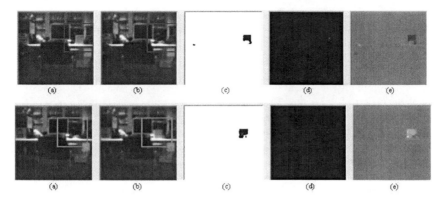

Fig. 4. (a) Background; (b) Image Flow; (c) Threshold; (d) Mass Centres; (e) Segmented Image

7 Conclusions

New services are possible using image-based sensors in AAL scenarios. These sensors enrich environment information which improves special services as User Tracking System, User Modelling System and Object Tracking System.

This paper presents some simple innovative image processing algorithms (Stolen-Abandoned Object Detection and Tracking People-Objects Algorithm) for autonomous vision sensors. Information treatment is done inside the sensor. In this way system increases its performance and avoid server processing and overload communications. Theses algorithms allow the implementation of AAL services, improving the user quality of life.

As future work, we are working in two new algorithms: a basic gestural interface (count the number of fingers and motion tracking), and a basic face recognition algorithm (works with low number of facial characteristics). These algorithms allow us to implement a lot of new AAL services, highlighting the need to include autonomous vision systems in AAL scenarios.

Acknowledgments. This work was funded by the Spanish Ministry of Industry, Tourism and Trade, under Research Grant TSI-020301-2009-18 (eCID), the Spanish Ministry of Science and Innovation, under Research Grant TEC2009-14595-C02-01, and the CENIT Project Segur@.

References

1. The Euser Project. eUser-Workpackage 1: Conceptual and Analytical Framework (Part A and Part C). In: European Commission. 6th Framework Programme. Contact number: IST-2002-507180 (2002)
2. Remagnino, P., Foresti, G.L.: Ambient Intelligence: A New Multidisciplinary Paradigm. IEEE Transactions on Systems, Man and Cybernetics, Part A 35(sup. 1), 1–6 (2005) ISSN: 1083-4427

3. Moya, J.M., et al.: AMISEC: Leveraging Redundancy and Adaptability to Secure AmI Applications. International Journal on Advances in Security. IARIA 1, 15–25 (2008)
4. Snidaro, L., Micheloni, C., Chiavedale, C.: Video Security for Ambient Intelligence. IEEE Transactions on Systems, Man and Cybernetics, Part A: Systems and Humans 35(1), 133–144 (2005) ISSN: 1083-4427
5. Karabiber, F., Arena, P., Fortuna, L., De Fiore, S., Vagliasindi, S., Arik, S.: Implementation of A Moving Target Tracking Algorithm Using Eye-RIS Vision System on A Mobile Robot. Journal of Signal Processing Systems (2010)
6. Sapuppo, F., Intaglietta, M., Bucolo, M.: Bio-Microfluidics Real-Time Monitoring Using CNN Technology. IEEE Transactions on Biomedical Circuits and Systems 2(2) (June 2008)
7. Gonzalez, R.C., Woods, R.E.: Digital Image Processing, 3rd edn. Pearson Prentice hall, London (2008) ISBN: 0-13-168728-x 978-0-13-168728-8
8. Araujo, A.: Metodología para el Desarrollo de Aplicaciones Basada en Servicios sobre Entornos Inteligentes. PhD. Thesis (May 2007)
9. Kobsa, A.: Generic User Modelling Systems. User Modelling and User-adapted Interaction 11(1-2), 49–63 (2001)
10. Anafocus: Eye-RIS Vision System Evaluation Kit. Hardware Description (2006)

A Methodology for Developing Accessible Mobile Platforms over Leading Devices for Visually Impaired People

Patricia Arroba, Juan Carlos Vallejo,
Álvaro Araujo, David Fraga, and José M. Moya

Dept. Ingeniería Electrónica
ETSI Telecomunicación
Universidad Politécnica de Madrid
{parroba,jcvallejo,araujo,dfraga,josem}@die.upm.es
http://www.elb105.es

Abstract. Mobile user interfaces are moving to new touchscreen technologies setting new barriers for the blind. Many solutions and designs have been proposed but none is complete for the vast heterogeneous variety of devices.

In this paper, we present a methodology for developing an accessible-to-blind platform based on the principles that visually impaired people should be able to access leading technology and no specific hardware should be necessary for it. Besides, our solution provides input and output methods adapted to any underlying hardware as proof of concept and a guidelines for developing mobile platforms and applications.

1 Introduction

In the last years, we are being witness to the huge increase of the number of smartphones. Apple sold near two million of iPhone 4^{TM} [1,2] before being released and Google activates 300,000 new Android^{TM}smartphones every day [3]. The main feature of these devices is the user experience increase by using touchscreens instead of buttons, trackballs and keyboards.

The strong evolution of the user experience and the Human-Computer Interaction (HCI) technologies forces people to rely more on visual cues and reduce the information received by the sense of touch. It presents a huge barrier to visual impaired users who are unable to access any feature of old and new technology. Basic actions such as a phone call are challenges that visually impaired people face everyday. This is even more serious if we consider that, according to the American Foundation for the Blind (AFB), only in USA, 25 million of people live with vision loss [4].

On the other hand, the Open Handset Alliance (OHA) was created to accelerate innovation in mobile and offer consumers a richer, less expensive, and better mobile experience [5]. The result is the first complete, open, and free mobile platform: Android^{TM}. However, for visually impaired users the platform is not as open and rich as the OHA intends to.

J. Bravo, R. Hervás, and V. Villarreal (Eds.): IWAAL 2011, LNCS 6693, pp. 209–215, 2011.

In this paper, we afford the challenge of completing such open mobile platform by making it accessible for every user. Organizations like AFB or the Spanish ONCE make an effort so visually impaired people can have access to the technology as well as the rest of the users.

Furthermore, according to these organizations, we will keep in mind the following principles:

- The visually impaired people should be able to access leading technology.
- That technology usage by the blind should be as closely matching it as the regular usage is. That means no specific hardware involved.

2   Related Work

Several solutions have been designed or, even, developed. In Vanderheiden [6] we can found the first approach to a screen reader but it needs a hardware button to confirm the actions.

WebAnywhere is a web-based, self-voicing browser that enables blind web users to access the web from almost any browser enabled device that can produce sound [7]. However, in spite of the web spread it is not a complete solution due to lots of existing native applications which are not based on the Web.

There are other partial solutions like No-Look Notes [8] which presents an alternative to the software keyboard. However, it has no haptic feedback and also provides no visual information about the text written, creating new barriers for the users with partial vision.

Also there exist complete solutions such as Slide Rule [9] and VoiceOver by Apple [10]. However, these ones are designed for working with hardware with specific characteristics. Particularly, VoiceOver only works on iPhone, iPad and iPod Touch and not every application is accessible but only the system core. On the other hand, Slide Rule has no visual feedback at all, preventing users with partial vision from see anything on the screen.

In summary, there are several solutions with limitations which hinders the access of the blind people to leading technology. So, our target is to design a global and accessible system within reach of every kind of user. Besides, during the design and development of the methods and tools proposed we have count on the help of CIDAT [11] experts which contributed testing and advise. In this paper he section 3 shows the considerations to make a system accessible. In section 4 we will see the gesture primitives and their usage in the system. The section 5 defines a low level specification. In section 6 we afford an accessible input text method development to demonstrate the feasibility of out work. Finally, in section 7 we show the results of the work.

3   Design Considerations

To achieve an accesibility platform, making it available to visual impaired users, we have developed a methodology that embraces a gestural user interface, that allows them to explore the information presented on the screen, and activate the different items. These items must have some specific resources that can be made accessible. Several consideration have been taken in order to achieve an accessible platform:

- Built in the device. Features like an accessibility service, sound and haptic feedback, screen orientation and speech rate should be selected from the device configuration screens. In this way, the device will not need any specific additional hardware.
- Provide a locale service. Changing the language of the device, will change locale features of the application, not having to rely on additional software.
- Intuitive gesture interface. The user interface must implement different gestures to quickly perform actions such as explore or activate screen items.
- Provide feedback to the user. The system should provide spoken, audible, and haptic feedback to describe the actions that have occurred.
- Handle options faster. The system should allow to perform any action with the less number of steps as possible.
- As fluently as needed. The users must be able to customize the features according to their needs and their improvement in the management of the application.

4   Accessibility Gestural Interface

The purpose looked for in this section is to examine a solution that associate a set of gestures to perform generic actions in order to make accessible gestural interfaces intuitive and easy to learn by visual impaired users. All these actions return a spoken feedback describing item features.

As we can see in Fig. 1, every gesture specified is available to any device with a touchscreen, whether it is multitouch or not. Therefore, there exist no gesture which uses more than two fingers. Two finger gestures are detected by monotouch screens by processing the area and the pressure of the gesture.

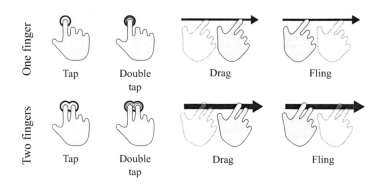

Fig. 1. Basic gestures with one and two fingers

Consequently, the main actions in which this methodology is focused are:

- **Focus and speech.** These actions are associated to navigation through the screen items. For each one the system will speak a brief description about the last focused item.
    - Drag over the screen: focus each item as the user passes his finger over it. The system will tell the last item focused.
    - Tap: focus the touched item.
    - Fling left: focus the next item.
    - Fling right: focus the previous item.
    - Fling down: focus the item below.
    - Fling up: focus the item above.
- **Activate.** Double tap anywhere on the screen activates the focused item. In this way, blind users would not need to locate again the focused item for activating it.
- **Complete speech.** The actions listed below are used to provide spoken feedback to the user about the complete set of items displayed on the screen.
    - Two fingers tap: stops the current feedback.
    - Two fingers double tap: report the number of items displayed on the screen.
    - Two fingers fling down: describes all the items from the focus.
    - Two fingers fling up: describes all the items displayed on the screen.
- **Scroll.** Moving through vertical and horizontal lists.
    - Tap and drag left/right: handles horizontal scrolling
    - Tap and drag down/up: handles vertical scrolling.
- **Seek bar.** To set the current progress the user may tap and drag in either directions on the item.
- **Display context menu.** Tap and long press on the screen shows the context menu in the foreground.

5   Low-Level Accessibility Resources

According to this methodology, a set of parameters will be required to return a spoken feedback, describing the features of the graphical items displayed on the screen. These resources may be enabled independently of each other in a configuration screen, so that the users can change these settings manually, to suit their skills. These parameters are listed below:

- Label: Word or brief phrase that characterizes each element displayed on the screen, providing identification.
- Summary: Resource that reports additional information on the use of the item. It will not be necessary in those items where the use is implied in their labels.
- Hint: Describes the action performed by activating the item.
- Position: Position of the focused item on the screen.
- Status: Provides information about system status changes.

- Value: Reports information about the current quantity, numerical amount or state for those items that require accurate data.

Therefore, every graphical item in a mobile platform should be able to provide these parameters in order to be completely accessible. Any application developed over that system will be accessible too.

6   Proof of Concept

In the previous sections we have establish a methodology and guidelines to create an accessible mobile platform. In order to analyze the feasibility of our work, this section will show an accessible software keyboard application developed by us and the instructions of how the user can interact with it.

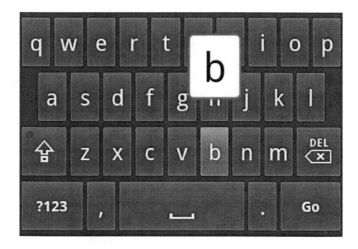

Fig. 2. Accessible software keyboard capture

Explore the user interface. Drag over the screen will allow the user to explore the keyboard without activate any key. In this way, the users will have feedback about each item as they touch it. Spoken feedback is a word or brief phrase that describes the pressed character and if it is capitalized. Moreover, the vibration of the device will indicate switching from one key to another, providing guidance to the user, unlike No-Look Notes [8].

Some characters such as vowels have special features. When pressure is maintained long on one of them, the user will open a keyboard that shows that vowel combined with the different accents and also a key to return without writing. The shift key causes a different speech depending on the state in which the keyboard was to inform the user when it is case sensitive. On the other hand, the symbols key indicates the type of keyboard that activates when you press it. No-Look Notes not allows the user to input symbols or special characters [8].

Character input. There are several methods to input data into an editable text box using this software keyboard such as lifting your finger from the screen on the key, double tap on the character and simultaneous multitouch on the key and another area of the screen off the keyboard. Switching between these input methods is done through a configuration screen associated to the keyboard. Otherwise, in Vanderheiden [6], a hardware button is needed to confirm all the actions.

Moreover, different characters have different features when introduced in the text box. By default, when the user enters a character, he can hear a distinctive sound followed by its description speech and confirmation by a slightly longer vibration. If the pressed key matches the character delete, when activated, the speech also contains the character that was deleted. Instead, if the written character is a space, a default confirmation is followed by a speech of the last written word in the text box.

Gesture input method. First of all, this gestures only work when the user performs on the software keyboard so none of them conflicts with other applications.

Some keys such as space or delete have an equivalent gesture in this accessible software keyboard. Performing a left fling will allow the user to delete the last character written faster. In the same way, a right fling will insert a space in the text box.

Finally, if the user flings up on the software keyboard, the full content of the editable text box is announced, indicating the cursor position in the edit text, reporting the user the information about the accurate location where he is entering text. If the user instead flings it down, the keyboard type is changed according to the features selected in the configuration screen.

7   Conclusions

We introduced a new methodology for developing accessible mobile platforms for devices with touchscreen input. The solutions is hardware independent so it can work on devices with screen supporting one touch or more. It lets visually impaired people use leading technology with no specific hardware.

The solution provides a functional gesture specification, a developing guidelines to make consistent mobile platforms and a customizable input application.

Acknowledgments

This work was supported by CIDAT (ONCE). Special thanks to Luis Palomares and Vanessa González.

References

1. The New York Times: Laptop sales help Apple top forecasts (2010),
   http://www.nytimes.com/2010/01/26/technology/companies/26appleearn.html

2. Hughes, N.: AppleInsider: Piper: 15.8M US iPhone sales in 2010, even without Verizon (2010), http://www.appleinsider.com/articles/10/01/06/piper_15_8m_us_iphone_sales_in_2010_even_without_verizon.html
3. Engadget: Andy Rubin: over 300,000 Android phones activated daily (2010), http://www.engadget.com/2010/12/09/andy-rubin-over-300-000-android-phones-activated-daily/
4. American Foundation for the Blind: Living with Vision Loss (2010), http://www.afb.org/
5. Open Handset Alliance (2010), http://www.openhandsetalliance.com/
6. Vanderheiden, G.C.: Use of Audio-Haptic Interface Techniques to Allow Nonvisual Access to Touchscreen Appliances. In: Human Factors and Ergonomics Society Annual Meeting Proceedings, vol. 40(1), pp. 1266–1266 (1996)
7. Bigham, J.P., Prince, C.M., Ladner, R.E.: WebAnywhere: a screen reader on-the-go. In: Proceedings of the 2008 International Cross-disciplinary Conference on Web Accessibility (W4A), pp. 73–82 (2008)
8. Bonner, M., Brudvik, J., Abowd, G., Edwards, W.: No-Look Notes: Accessible Eyes-Free Multi-touch Text Entry. Pervasive Computing, 409–426 (2010)
9. Kane, S.K., Bigham, J.P., Wobbrock, J.O.: Slide rule: making mobile touch screens accessible to blind people using multi-touch interaction techniques. In: Proceedings of the 10th International ACM SIGACCESS Conference on Computers and Accessibility, pp. 73–80 (2010)
10. Apple, Inc.: VoiceOver: Accessibility solution for iPhone (2010), http://www.apple.com/accessibility/iphone/vision.htm
11. ONCE: Centro de Investigación, Desarrollo y Aplicación Tiflotécnica, http://cidat.once.es

Context-Awareness as an Enhancement of Brain-Computer Interfaces

Agustin A. Navarro[1], Luigi Ceccaroni[1], Filip Velickovski[1], Sergi Torrellas[1],
Felip Miralles[1], Brendan Z. Allison[2], Reinhold Scherer[2], and Josef Faller[2]

[1] Barcelona Digital Technology Centre, Roc Boronat 117, 08018 Barcelona, Spain
{anavarro,lceccaroni,fvelickovski,storrellas,
fmiralles}@bdigital.org
[2] Laboratory of Brain-Computer Interfaces, Graz University of Technology, Krenngasse 37,
8010 Graz, Austria
{allison,reinhold.scherer,josef.faller}@tugraz.at

Abstract. Ambient intelligence has acquired a relevant presence in assistive technologies. Context-awareness, the ability to perceive situations and to act providing suitable responses, plays a key role in such presence. BrainAble, an ongoing European project, aims at raising the autonomy of people with functional diversity, facilitating and enhancing the interaction with their environment. Brain-computer interfaces are applied as communication means to allow users to perform actions by using their electroencephalogram signals. Multiple approaches are studied and combined in order to provide the best set of brain signals which specifies a concrete event or action. In this setting, we propose the application of context-awareness to extend the traditional proactive and pervasive nature of ambient intelligence in a way which enhances the brain-computer interface. One practical example is the dynamic personalization of available options in the user interface, based on user's current context.

Keywords: Assisted Living, Brain-Computer Interfaces, Context-Awareness, Contextual Facilitation.

1 Introduction

Ambient intelligence (AmI) has introduced a new source of potential applications and services with a promising impact on assistive technologies. The role of AmI is generally related to the home automation or control of ubiquitous devices in the environment. However, the AmI feature that provides the most benefits in terms of assistance to the users is its context-awareness, which, in the case of assistive technologies, refers to the recognition of situations and acting according to the level of assistance required.

Systems that can represent and process information about context can address special requirements of the ageing society and people with functional diversity, and can personalize tasks and support software-tools according to the needs and situations of each individual. Thus, AmI could assist people with functional diversity in their daily life to improve their autonomy and living conditions. Approaches that rely on

J. Bravo, R. Hervás, and V. Villarreal (Eds.): IWAAL 2011, LNCS 6693, pp. 216–223, 2011.

this type of technology to accomplish assistive tasks have been mainly focused on the monitoring and recognition of *activities of daily life* (ADLs). For example, one approach detects complex human activities from a continuous sequence of events to prevent emergencies [1]. Another example is the implementation of a multi-agent architecture (connecting healthcare institutions, patients and their relatives on a common network) for monitoring and recognizing specific situations [2]. Similarly, a rehabilitation approach was designed to provide users with topographical disorientation with adaptive tools and feedback based on their own actions [3].

Brainable, an ongoing project funded by the European Commission (FP7 grant agreement n° 247447), aims to improve quality of life among people with functional diversities by overcoming two of the main shortcomings they suffer: exclusion from home activities and social activities. The main objectives are therefore the enhancement of their autonomy and independency for ADLs, and the improvement of their social inclusion. Within the project, the achievement of these objectives strongly relies on the use of *brain-computer interfaces* (BCIs), which are systems that allow communication and control via thought alone [4] [5] [6]. They are based on the direct measures of brain activity and are employed in conjunction with other technologies such as AmI, social networking and virtual reality. Thereby, users are empowered to take actions or express their desires in the form of decisions selected from a set of options supplied by a user interface.

The role of AmI over the provision of control capabilities to the user is mainly to carry out the interaction with the real environment by performing the user's commands (e.g., to turn on a light). In addition, an unobtrusive network of pervasive devices acts to proactively manage emergency, security, comfort or energy-saving issues. Thanks to context-awareness, specific situations are recognized and suitable responses are performed.

A number of BCI approaches have been heavily researched and rely on different recording methods, modes of operation and mental strategies to obtain specific patterns of activity. In any case, they are limited and cannot compete with natural communications or traditional human-computer interfaces in most situations [7]. In this paper, we address issues in incorporating context-awareness to enhance BCI performance. Thus, considering this type of aid as a contextual facilitation, it could be stated that if BCI is a bottom-up, stimulus-driven perceptual mechanism, then context is its top-down inference complement.

The remainder of the paper, Sections 2 and 3, provide a background for the Brainable project, as well as the features and constraints of BCI. Section 4 introduces context-awareness as an enhancement of BCI and its corresponding benefits for the user, and Section 5 describes the architecture and its implementation in the first prototype of the Brainable platform. This is followed by a description of future work and some concluding remarks.

2   The Brainable Project

It is known that motor functional diversity of any source have a dramatic effect on people's quality of life. The Brainable project addresses this problem from several perspectives. It conceives, researches, designs, implements and validates a *human-computer interface* (HCI) composed of BCI sensors combined with affective computing. These technologies aim at improving the quality of life of people suffering from functional diversity by addressing their two major limitations: exclusion from home and social activities. Brainable operates in the inner world for functional independence for ADLs and in the outer world for social inclusion. The project's platform helps then people with functional diversity manage their living environment and improve social interaction.

Objectives of Brainable's user-centric platform are: (1) to improve the quality of life of people with motor functional diversity, (2) to increase autonomy in ADLs and social inclusion, (3) to decrease communication barriers, (4) to create a specifically designed HCI, which integrates BCI with other specific sensor technologies, (5) to build user-centric virtual environments for home and urban automation control, social networking and training, (6) to create AmI and ubiquitous-computing services for accessible device integration, by adapting a *universal remote console* (URC) / UCH standard platform and (7) to investigate self-expression media, VR-based tools and social networking services in relation to BCIs.

Brainable expects to build and test a product prototype and a set of associated technologies intended to assist people with physical functional diversity ranging from speech disorders to *motor neuron disease* to *locked-in syndrome*. It will facilitate the management of networks of interoperable devices and the access to computer-based social networks for better inclusion.

3   Brain-Computer Interfaces

A BCI is a novel means of communication. Sometimes called a *direct neural interface* or a *brain-machine interface*, it is a direct communication pathway between a human brain and an external device. In Brainable, BCI development is based on the non-invasive electroencephalogram (EEG). EEG signals are potential differences recorded from electrodes placed on the scalp and reflect the temporal and spatial summation of electrical inputs to large groups of neurons lying beneath the recording electrode. BCIs have a very limited bandwidth and cannot compete with other means such as speaking, writing or traditional HCIs [7], but can be extremely useful for users who cannot speak, write or use traditional HCIs. The main problem with BCIs is the poor *information transfer rate* (ITR), which is the amount of information a user can send in a certain interval, and is expressed in bits per units of time. ITR may be used to measure performance in BCIs or other communication systems, and relies on three factors: the number of available signals or commands (N), the accuracy in classifying the desired signal (P), and the number of signals per minute (S) [4].

Early BCI research efforts focused primarily on proving that a system could work, and then on validating BCIs with patients and field settings. While these are critical goals, early work did not consider how to incorporate context. That is, a BCI signal was translated into a message or command regardless of contextual information such as recent commands, available options, or the state of the user or system.

This has begun to change, with increasing attention to goal-oriented protocols and context-aware BCIs in more recent work [6] [8]. Thus by adding contextual information could increase the effective ITR of a BCI by allowing users to accomplish their goals more quickly and effectively. A system that only allows a user to convey 10 bits per minute may be quite adequate for many needs if the user does not need to painstakingly communicate unnecessary details.

4 Contextual Facilitation

In Brainable, BCI communication acquires an especially significant importance, because it enables people with severe functional diversities to interact with their environment. As mentioned above, considering its limitations, BCI performance may be enhanced by using context-awareness as complement. To better understand this complementarity, let us consider the analogy of language processing, which is also strongly influenced by context. According to the two major psycholinguistic hypotheses which analyse the linguistic interplay, there are two distinct mechanisms: a bottom-up one, sensitive to linguistic information and a top-down one, sensitive to contextual knowledge [9]. According to the Gradient Salience hypothesis [10], these two mechanisms run in parallel and interact in order to foster language comprehension. A related comparison was explored in [8]. In this paper, Wolpaw noted that the human body relies on top-down, high level processes and bottom-up, low-level processes. People may decide to get a glass of water, and then initiate a process with many low-level details that are not consciously processed. People do not think about how exactly to move their legs or coordinate visual stimuli (such as the location of a glass) with motor activity (such as pouring into the glass). The paper notes that BCIs should be similar. BCI users should not have to inform a robotic arm of all the necessary movement details. Instead, BCI users should be able to send one high-level command, such as "get water", and rely on the software to manage the lower-level details. Ideally, users should be presented with both high-level and low-level commands, so they can attain goals quickly if desired, but can also change medium or low-level details (such as getting juice instead of water, using a different cup, or avoiding the use of one finger that is injured.

Contextual facilitation may be therefore a complementary expectation-driven mechanism, which improves BCI performance by predicting oncoming events and by constraining and personalising possible options for the user to select. Two of the main research approaches to be applied in the Brainable project are the BCI improvement by personalization and by inference. Personalization refers to the dynamic presentation of the most convenient options to select from the user interface based on the current context, while inference refers to the presentation of predicted options based on user's preferences under a determined context.

Personalization could be useful in various contexts. In a smart home environment, a context aware system might know that a door is open, and thus would not present the user with the option of opening that door. In a smart home or VR environment, if a wheelchair, mobile robot, or virtual avatar is in front of a wall or other obstacle, then the option to move forward should not be available to the user [6] [8].

5 BrainAble's AmI Centric Architecture

Brainable is designed with a centralized modular architecture around the Ambient Intelligence (AmI) module. Fig. 1 shows a high level block diagram of the modules. It

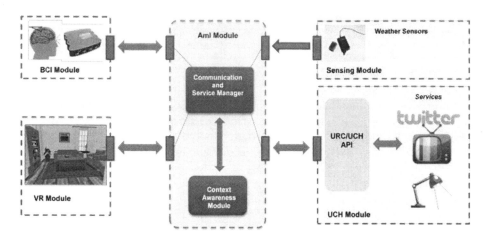

Fig. 1. Brainable centralized architecture consisting of 5 modules: *BCI Module, VR Module, Weather Sensors, UCH Module, AmI Module*

is composed of 5 modules: *BCI Module, VR Module, Weather Sensors, UCH Module, AmI Module*. Communication paths are shown as uni or bidirectional arrows and all communication paths in Brainable need to pass through the AmI Module.

BCI Module Contains the BCI processing logic, hardware, and GUI to transform the user's brain signals into an action or command to be executed. The BCI actions are accessed via a hierarchical menu that is visually presented to the user. For example the user must select using the BCI "Devices then TV then Channel 5" in order to execute the command that changes the channel on the television. The platform has been implemented with two BCI GUIs, the P300 Matrix [11] and Hex-o-Select [12]. Selection in the BCI menu takes time, and selection of an action item takes even longer if it is embedded deep within the menu. Providing a context sensitive shortcut area in the BCI that is sensitive to context can reduce the number of selection considerably.

Sensing Module In order to gather useful contextual information, the sensing module will provide access to environmental and physiological sensors. Currently the room temperature, luminosity and humidity are being captured.

UCH Module The Universal Control Hub is a middleware to provide a uniform and consistent API to all devices and services via a HTTP protocol gateway. Devices can be attached to the UCH and their status and control are available via the gateway.

VR Module Brainable provides a virtually interactive environment for training a new user to the platform, and also for providing an enhanced experience. The user is represented by a virtual avatar and is able to navigate the virtual environment.

AmI Module All commands issued by the BCI pass through the AmI Module, and the sensor information also is relayed to this module. By continuous use of the system the AmI Module is able to learn the user's personal habits by a Bayesian based algorithm described later in the section. When a similar context arises, that is similar to one seen before, the AmI Module is able to provide back to the BCI a list of probabilities of the most likely actions. Using this list the BCI is able to provide through an adaptive shortcut area direct access to the action, saving the user time spent by navigating through the hierarchical menu.

Services in Brainable Prototype

In the first prototype the limited services included are listed in Table 1 along with the corresponding actions that are selectable in the BCI menu.

Table 1. Table of services with actions offered in Brainable prototype

Service Type	Service	Actions
Domotic device	Light	On, Off
	TV	On, Off, Set Channel (1..5), Volume Up, Volume Down
Social	Twitter	Log On, Log Off Send Tweet, Get Tweets

Context

Context in [13] is defined as any information that can be used to characterize the situation of an entity. In Brainable it is captured by a list of Boolean, and numeric descriptors that are gathered via the sensors (temperature, humidity, luminosity), the service states (light, tv, twitter login status) and the current time (day of the week, hour of the day, season).

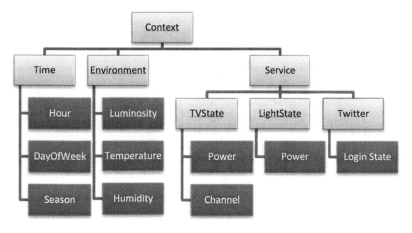

Fig. 2. Context consists of a set of descriptors (leaf nodes) from time, environment sensors and service status

These inputs are shown in Fig. 2 as the leaf nodes, the upper nodes reveal the category the context descriptor belongs to. The descriptors allow the AmI Module to characterize a particular situation, for example: it is late at night on the weekend, and the user is watching TV, on channel 4, while the light is turned off. In the next section we present how using a Bayesian approach the AmI Module can learn to anticipate action from the context.

Learning from Context

In order to address the slow selection speed of the BCI we proposed to use the user's context to anticipate the most likely actions, furthermore these actions could be presented in an adaptive shortcut area of the BCI menu so that the user does not have to waste time by navigating through the menu hierarchy, instead the action is available more directly in the shortcut area available at all times in the BCI GUI.

An effective and well studied Bayesian classifier is Naive Bayes [14]. It is capable of estimating probabilities for classes after training with a set of features, and has already proved effective in context classification from sensor based networks [15]. In our case, we use this method to obtain an estimate for $P(A / Context)$ where A is an actions listed in Table 1 and $Context = \{X_1, X_2, X_3...X_n\}$ are the context descriptors of Fig. 2. The context descriptors that are continuous, such as luminosity, are quantized into a discrete number of values so that statistics can be counted. Finally the probability can then be estimated using the Bayes rule and the statistical independent naive assumption:

$$P(A|X_1,X_2,X_3...X_n) = P(A) \, P(X_1|A) \, P(X_2|A) \, ... \, P(X_n|A) \, Z \qquad (1)$$

Where $P(A)$ and $P(X_i/A)$ represent the prior probability, and conditional probability, both calculated during training, and Z is the normalizing factor.

Training occurs automatically and is personalized to the user by the continued use of the Brainable system. All commands are routed through the AmI Module and it keeps a record of statistics in histograms of each action against each context descriptor in order to calculate the conditional probabilities $P(X_i/A)$ needed. Eventually the system will capture patterns that emerge about the user's personal habits. For example the user turns on the light everyday when the luminosity falls below a certain value, or the user turns on the TV on weekends at 8pm. The next time this context is encountered the adaptive BCI interface will offer the appropriate action directly as equation (1) will produce a high probability for these actions.

6 Conclusions and Future Work

The Brainable project is in an early stage where a first integration of technologies to satisfy user requirements has resulted in a 1st Year Prototype. Validating the ideas in the Brainable project requires additional development, implementation, testing, and revision. The Brainable consortium plans to study and assess different BCI mental strategies and their combination with other physiological signals to assess their feasibility. There are different options on how to apply contextual facilitation. This paper presented some possibilities, but some other options are also worth exploring. In addition, context awareness presents different challenges across different input signals, users, devices, applications, and environments. The objective is to assess and learn from these early approaches in order to improve and implement these innovative ideas on suitable assisting services.

References

1. Prueckner, S., Madler, C., Beyer, D., Berger, M., Kleinberger, T., Becker, T.: Emergency Monitoring and Prevention – EU Project EMERGE. In: Proc. Ambient Assisted Living (2008)
2. Carneiro, D., Costa, R., Novais, P., Machado, J., Neves, J.: Simulating and Monitoring Ambient Assisted Living. In: Proc. ESM (2008)
3. Morganti, F.: Riva. G.: Ambient Intelligence for Rehabilitation. In: Riva, G., Vatalaro, F., Davide, F., Alcañiz, M. (eds.), IOS Press, Amsterdam (2005)
4. Wolpaw, J.R., Birbaumer, N., McFarland, D.J., Pfurtscheller, G., Vaughan, T.M.: Brain-Computer Interfaces for Communication and Control. Clinical Neurophysiology 113 (2002)
5. Pfurtscheller, G., Müller-Putz, G.R., Schlögl, A., Graimann, B., Scherer, R., Leeb, R., Brunner, C., Keinrath, C., Lee, F., Townsend, G., Vidaurre, C., Neuper, C.: 15 years of BCI research at Graz University of Technology: current projects. IEEE Trans. Neural Systems and Rehabilitation Engineering 14, 205–210 (2006)
6. Allison, B.Z., Wolpaw, E.W., Wolpaw, J.R.: Brain computer interface systems: Progress and prospects. In: Poll, E. (ed.) British Review of Medical Devices, vol. 4(4), pp. 463–474 (July 2007)
7. Graimann, B., Allison, B., Pfurtscheller, G.: Brain-Computer Interfaces: Revolutionizing Human-Computer Interaction, 1st edn. Springer, Heidelberg (2010)
8. Wolpaw, J.R.: Brain-computer Interfaces as new Brain Output Pathways. J. Physiol. (2007)
9. Kecskes, I.: On My Mind: Thoughts about Salience, Context and Figurative Language from a Second Language Perspective. Second Language Research 22, 2 (2006)
10. Peleg, O., Giora, R., Fein, O.: Salience and Context Effects: Two are Better than One. Metaphor. & Symbol 16, 173–192 (2001)
11. Donchin, E., Spencer, K.M., Wijesinghe, R.: The Mental Prosthesis: Assessing the Speed of a P300-Based Brain-Computer Interface. IEEE Trans. Rehab. Eng. 8(2), 174–179 (2000)
12. Blankertz, B., Dornhege, G., Krauledat, M., Schröder, M., Williamson, J., Murray-Smith, R., Müller, K.R.: The Berlin Brain-Computer Interface Presents the Novel Mental Typewriter Hex-O-Spell. In: 3rd Int. BCO Work. And Training Course, Graz (2006)
13. Dey, A.K.: Understanding and using context. Personal and Ubiquitous Computing 5, 20–24 (2001)
14. Theodoridis, S., Koutroumbas, T.: Pattern Recognition, 4th edn. Elsevier, Amsterdam (2009)
15. Korpipää, P., Koskinen, M., Peltola, J.: Bayesian Approach to Sensor-Based Context Awareness. Pers. Ubiquitous Computing 7, 113–124 (2003)

Author Index